LOSE TEN YEARS IN TEN DAYS

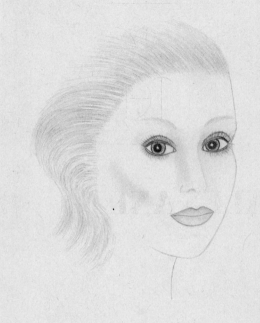

LOSE TEN YEARS IN TEN DAYS

ALEXANDRA YORK

MACMILLAN PUBLISHING CO., INC. □ NEW YORK

Macmillan Publishing Co., Inc.
866 Third Avenue, New York, N.Y. 10022
Collier Macmillan Canada, Ltd.

Library of Congress Cataloging in Publication Data
York, Alexandra.
Lose ten years in ten days.
Includes index.
1. Beauty, Personal.   2. Middle-aged women—
Health and hygiene.   I. Title.
RA778.Y56   646.7′2′0880564   80-28038
ISBN 0-02-633270-1

10 9 8 7 6 5 4 3 2 1

Printed in the United States of America

ILLUSTRATIONS BY DIANE CRESTON

To the self-made woman

CONTENTS

INTRODUCTION

Yes you can. In fact, losing ten *years* is both faster and easier than losing ten *pounds*. Most women look their age—and up to ten years older—for two main reasons. Number one is simple neglect. Number two (and more important) is lack of individuality.

Consider the easiest first. Neglect. Most excuses for letting oneself go usually claim a lack of time. "I never have time for myself because of _____." In the blank space insert your own excuse: children, your career, your husband's career, social responsibilities, ill parents. . . . It really doesn't matter which excuse you offer, because most likely none of them is valid. We all know that time can be found for anything we *want* to do. The true reason behind neglect of our personal selves is almost always a much more uncommendable culprit, recognized as an old, unfriendly friend to many women and men alike—laziness.

The scenario often goes like this: First, you stop really bothering with makeup; a little foundation and a drop of lipstick begin to make do. Next, rather than putting together a clothes look each day, you grab what's cleanest or throw on a pair of pants and a shirt or sweater. Undoubtedly, one of the greatest reasons blue jeans became and stayed so popular for so long was pure laziness. It takes no thought to pull on the same pants day after day, the only difference being their state of cleanliness. Last on the list of neglected items goes the body, and when that goes, so eventually goes an inner energy for imaginative (young) living.

Laziness may also take another rather surprising form, which, once translated, is simply a hidden excuse for neglecting one's appearance. I have had very stylish women tell me that they have been accused by their friends (less stylish, of course) of taking *too* much care of themselves and looking *too good!* They have been accused of being vain, selfish and self-centered. Now, if you are one of these maligned women, the problem is not yours. It is perfectly proper to make the very best of one's appearance. It is perfectly proper to be selfish; this whole book is devoted to helping you become even more so. The benefits to be gained from self-attention range all the way from feeling better about yourself (as you look better), to getting better service (good looks attract attention), to getting elected to an office.

If some friend of yours is trying to get you to become as lazy as she is by deprecating your efforts, don't listen to a word. And if you are that friend, it is *you* who should pull yourself up out of the laziness that causes you to criticize others.

Beyond laziness in whatever disguise it may appear, a second, and more fundamental, factor contributing to "age gain" is failure to conceptualize an individual look. We are an ever-changing phenomenon; whether or not we consciously acknowledge this fact does not alter the truth of it. The human experience does not stand still. And time does not stand still. Wearing the clothes and makeup of your own youth or, worse, copying the fads of the young today, only adds years to your appearance because the contrast between you and your attempts is so obvious. Following fashion fads in general emphasizes anyone's age, in fact, because it focuses an observer's attention on how the latest fad (or more often one that has already passed) looks on you—at your age—rather than on how *you* look.

If you neither follow fads nor try to dress younger than you are and continue to look older than you would like to, the reason is usually still lack of individuality, but in another form—conventionality. As an experiment, visit your regular supermarket, department store or shopping center, strictly as an observer. Not an observer of goods to buy, but of the people buying them. Notice their clothes, their hairstyles, their purses, their shoes. Does everybody look pretty much alike? Do you look, generally speaking, pretty much like most of them? If you do, then you have allowed your appearance to change gradually (unthinkingly) along with the most commonly adopted dress, makeup and hairstyle behavior of the masses, which also emphasizes your age because it usually doesn't really suit *you*.

The only way to circumvent the whole subject of age in your outward appearance is to express your own individuality by your external dress and beauty choices. And since you are an ever-changing human being, it is necessary to become consciously aware of your continuing *growth*—not your continuing *age*—and adjust your appearance accordingly.

Luckily, you can get rid of both a boring appearance and up to ten years in age, whatever your particular reason for gaining them, in just a few days of concentrated effort. And it can even be fun. The happy truth is—and I have seen it happen many times in my beauty seminars —that in only ten short days you can give a real "face-lift" not only to your face, but to your wardrobe and mind as well. An altogether younger you. You'll feel it on the inside, and you won't be the only one to notice it on the outside.

Think of this ten-day program as an age diet. Each day you lose another year. Or, if this image is more helpful, think of it as a personal training program. Because that's precisely what it is. You'll be *re*training your normal, habitual beauty habits to change them or freshen them and bring them up to date. Not up to date according to indications from fashion magazines and display windows, but up to date in relation to your own growth patterns, your own life-style, your own values . . . your own identity.

The activities have been arranged so that you may devote many hours to this program or just squeeze the time in along with your normal schedule. Be prepared, because you are going to be busy, but the amount of time you invest in this program is not what make these ideas work; it's the mental focus and the real insistence on accomplishing all of the activities each day that really count. If you are not employed, you can do the A.M. activities in the morning and the P.M. in the afternoon. If you work or have other nonadjustable schedules, you can get up early for the A.M. activities and do the P.M. after work or in the evening, slipping any shopping called for into your lunch hour. The crucial element is to *do* each day's activities on the day scheduled, *each* day, *consecutively*. On a short, action-packed, ten-day program, if you skip a day of two, don't expect results. But if you commit yourself, as if in a training program, to the full ten-day regime, the results will really be astonishing. Ten days, surely, isn't a long time. One of the reasons twenty-one-day programs usually fail is that the time span is too long.

Who can realistically spend that much time? But ten days, even squeezed into your normal routine . . . yes, you can.

There is one condition to this age diet. Don't tell anyone you are on it. If you do, talk can too easily replace action. Don't even go on this program with a friend. You'll only dilute each other's determination, you'll end up chatting about it instead of doing it, you'll unduly influence each other's taste and opinions, and if one of you looks better sooner, the other could lose her enthusiasm. So go on this diet alone. This is between you and you. For you. Don't even tell your family if you can help it. Do something, for a change, *for* yourself, *by* yourself. Afterward, as you go on looking better week after week—because if you do all that this book suggests for ten days, you won't likely give it all up as soon as the ten days are over—then you can tell everybody on the block. But by then, you won't have to say a word. They'll be asking you.

For now, however, only read on, concentrate on accomplishing everything on each day's list on the day specified. Don't worry about the time —it doesn't take that much. And don't worry about the money. If you scan the next few pages, you will see a lot of "go shopping for. . . ." But as you get into the program, you'll see that most of the time, shopping isn't to buy but to learn. And when I do suggest that you buy certain items for the program, they are only the things you should have been buying all along for your health and beauty care. I also adjust for every possible pocketbook, even if it's just about empty.

So don't worry. In fact, stop worrying about everything and just enjoy the next ten days. And ever after too . . . of course.

ALEXANDRA YORK

LOSE TEN YEARS IN TEN DAYS

DAY ONE

Do not panic! Today is a *much* busier day than usual. Because it is the first day, there are a certain number of start-up things to do. If it will help, do a few of the items the night before you start, such as reading the chapters indicated. If you are really pressed for time, you could begin the program on a weekend, using both Saturday and Sunday as Day One.

A.M.

STEP ONE

Hang over the side of the bed from the waist up and let the blood bring oxygen and energy to both your body and brain. Next, lie back flat in bed and stretch your body. Hands over your head, imagine that something is pulling you from opposite ends, one force pulling your hands and another pulling your feet. Begin each day of the program in this manner. Get up. Good morning.

1

STEP TWO

(Steps Two and Three may be reversed each day if you like.)

Breakfast—the same each day:

½ grapefruit
1 slice protein toast, dry (may be omitted)
1 multivitamin
1 cup coffee or tea (as you like it)

Eat sitting down at a table, and never again eat any future meal either standing up in the kitchen or while accomplishing some small task. *Taste* your food and give it a chance to digest properly. (After today, you will do your wake-up warm-ups before breakfast.)

STEP THREE

Shower or bathe.

Stand nude in front of a full-length mirror. If you don't have one, buy one. *No one* can expect to take or keep control of her appearance without regularly viewing herself from top to bottom. (If money is a factor, you can get a perfectly suitable mirror at the five-and-ten for under $10.)

Examine your body honestly. How long has it been since you have actually looked at it naked like this? Look at it now. Notice the way in which you hold your shoulders. The slope of your breasts. The width of your waist. The firmness of your hips and thighs. The size of your upper arms. Turn around. Check the size and firmness of your fanny.

Turn back to the side and then the front again, noticing only your posture. Many a woman can lose a few years instantaneously just by standing up straight. When you view your body from the side, see if the small of your back is basically flat and straight or if you seem to be standing swaybacked, with an arch in the small of your back and the stomach protruding. When viewing frontally, check to see if your shoulders are drooping to one side and if your waist seems to disappear into your hips.

Now, lift your shoulders up as far as you can and try to touch them to your ears. Holding that lifted position, press them back as far as they will go and then drop them into their natural, proper place. Lift your waist up out of your hips and tuck your pelvis under. In order to accomplish this, think of a string attached to the pelvic area and think of that string as being pulled forward—it is the *buttocks* you are pulling under and forward, not your hips. Lastly, pretend you have a dime to hold in the crack between your buttocks. Don't laugh, it works. During the day, remember that image and you'll see just how relaxed you've allowed your derrière to become, which then leads to the swayback, the stomach relaxing forward to compensate and the shoulders dropping to help the stomach. No matter what your weight, stand tall and you will drop years automatically.

Note down in the space provided in chapter 13—"Work Sheets"—three, and only three, areas that need attention . . . either toning, slimming, or filling out.

STEP FOUR

Dress and read chapters 1, 2, and 3 of this book.

STEP FIVE

Make a list of the ingredients you will need to make:

1 cleansing cream
1 skin freshener
1 moisturizing or protection cream
1 defoliating beauty mask

P.M.

STEP ONE

Go shopping for:

1. the ingredients you will need for your skin-care products
2. the ingredients for the following "health drink" (this will be your lunch each day):

—2 8-ounce containers plain yogurt
—1 quart skim milk
—eggs
—1 jar wheat germ
—1 package all-bran cereal (no additives, no preservatives)
—1 small box powdered milk
—1 small jar blackstrap molasses
—your choice of a container of fresh or frozen (without syrup) strawberries or two ripe bananas (my favorite) or one can of unsweetened pineapple chunks
—1 small can or jar brewer's yeast or, if you don't like the taste—I don't—one jar yeast tablets at the health food store .

3. 10 quart bottles of either sparkling or still mineral water or pure spring water of your choice (this is for sipping throughout each day—1 quart a day at your leisure).

STEP TWO

Call a *new* (this is important) hairdresser and make an appointment for the A.M. of the seventh day.

STEP THREE

Make creams and lotions for skin-care products.

STEP FOUR

Make fruit malted health drink in your blender and put in refrigerator:

Fruit Malted Health Drink

Mix together in blender:

> 2 *8-ounce containers plain yogurt*
> 1 *cup skim milk*
> 2 *eggs*
> ¼ *cup wheat germ*
> ¼ *cup all-bran cereal*
> ¼ *cup powdered milk*
> 1 *heaping tablespoon molasses*
> 1 *cup strawberries or two bananas or 1 cup*
>   *pineapple chunks*
> 1 *tablespoon brewer's yeast or take two yeast*
>   *tablets each time you drink this malted*

Taste. If the flavor is not sweet enough, add some honey or artificial sweetener until it is. You should *enjoy* this drink as a treat—it is not medicine. This is your lunch for the next nine days. *One 8-ounce glass each day.* When you run out, make another batch of a different flavor.

Note: There are no restrictions for dinners on this program. However, I suggest you eat simple, well-balanced meals and, if you must drink alcohol, no hard liquor and no more than one or two small glasses of wine per day.

STEP FIVE

Go to bed at an hour that will give you no more than eight hours' sleep.

DAY TWO

A.M.

STEP ONE

Morning stretch routine in bed as outlined in Day One. Turn to chapter 4 and perform morning wake-up warm-ups as outlined, plus spot exercises for the three areas you have chosen for special attention (this need not take more than ten or fifteen minutes).

STEP TWO

Breakfast.

STEP THREE

Shower or bathe.

STEP FOUR

Give yourself a defoliating facial according to the instructions in chapter 2.

Lunch

one 8-ounce glass of Fruit Malted (can be
transported easily in a Thermos bottle)

*Note: Don't forget your quart of mineral or spring water throughout the
day.*

P.M.

STEP ONE

Read chapter 5 on makeup.

STEP TWO

Go shopping for:

1.
1 new color of eyeshadow
1 brown or gray eyeliner (if you don't already have it)
1 medium-brown eye shadow (for accenting eyes and especially for
contouring face)
1 new lipstick
1 foundation (if you don't already have the proper shade)
any other products you wish

It makes no difference whether you shop at a ritzy department store
or at the dime store. Just be sure to go to the ritzy department store first
to play and experiment with colors, etc. Don't be embarrassed if you
don't buy anything there—merely say you want to live with whatever
you're trying for a while, smile and leave. Then, if you wish, purchase
the same color in a cheaper brand elsewhere.

2. three to five fashion magazines of your choice plus one home-
decorating magazine

DAY THREE

A.M.

STEP ONE

Morning stretch, morning wake-up warm-ups, plus exercises for three special-attention spots, breakfast, shower or bath and add your daily skin-care routine from chapter 2 (you will use this skin-care routine each day, once in the morning and again before bed).

STEP TWO

Apply makeup according to instructions in chapter 5.

Lunch

one 8-ounce glass of Fruit Malted

Note: Don't forget to sip your mineral or spring water.

P.M.

STEP ONE

At your leisure and without any predetermined thought or purpose, leaf through the fashion and decorating magazines you have purchased.

7

Simply cut out anything at all that strikes your fancy, whether it be a dress, a makeup look, a haircut, a room setting, a tree, a perfume ad, a flower, a car, a color. Don't even give one thought as to whether the subject is something you would actually want or could afford if you did want it, or whether you think the object is right for you. Don't think at all—it makes no difference. If you like it, even if you don't know why, cut it out. Put all clippings in a big envelope and set aside.

DAY FOUR

A.M.

STEP ONE

Morning stretch, morning wake-up warm-ups, plus exercises for three special-attention spots, breakfast, shower or bath, daily skin-care routine, daily makeup (Do *not* omit your daily makeup no matter what the rest of your day may be like—even if you're only going to see the mailman!).

STEP TWO

Read chapter 6 and compile your magic scrapbook.

Lunch

one 8-ounce glass of Fruit Malted

P.M.

STEP ONE

Go shopping for:
Clothes. Not to buy, but to experiment with the new style (or redefined old style) you have discovered as a result of your magic scrapbook.

9

Go to the best stores in your town, whether or not you can actually afford to buy there. Look at the most expensive clothes. Forget price; you are there to learn, not buy. After you experiment and become familiar with finely made clothes and good fabrics, you can select more wisely from cheaper copies. Don't feel intimidated by any salesclerk working in these expensive stores. Remember that most of the clerks working there can't afford to buy there either. Have fun. Don't be afraid of mistakes. Keep an open mind. Play.

STEP TWO

Read chapter 7 on signature hair.

Note: Don't forget your mineral or spring water.

DAY FIVE

A.M.

STEP ONE

Morning stretch, morning wake-up warm-ups, plus exercises for three special-attention spots, breakfast, shower or bath, daily skin-care routine, daily makeup. Dress well today, but select something that leaves you rather uncluttered around the neck area.

STEP TWO

Go shopping for:

Wigs. Not to buy, but to experiment with new hairstyles and colors. Try on many different styles (be open-minded—try long, short, curly, straight) to see which one will suit you and your *real* hair best. Try new colors, too. Even if you have had brown hair all your life or if you have tinted your hair red for fifteen years, experiment with colors as well. Your complexion has undoubtedly changed somewhat, and you may have chosen (or been born with) the wrong color hair for you as you are now. There is no need to explain to the salesperson the purpose of your visit.

11

Lunch

one 8-ounce glass of Fruit Malted

P.M.

STEP ONE

Go through all of your clothes closets and *ruthlessly* weed them. Set aside clothes to be given away (be brave) because they no longer express your individual style. Try on the rest to see if and how they might be altered to better suit the newly defined knowledge learned from your scrapbook. Be imaginative. Think of taking the lovely fabric from a dress that is not right for you and making it into a blouse. Shorten an evening gown into a dress. Take the top and sleeves off a dress and make it strapless. Keep only the jacket of a suit and use it as a blazer; try a belt with it. Turn a long gown into a hostess skirt.

Some of you may feel the desire, at this particular point, to seek some help from a friend. Don't do it! Following the judgment of others (even subconsciously) is part of the reason you need to lose ten years. Do the best you can—but do it alone. You may learn something about yourself that you didn't know before. Give yourself this chance.

STEP TWO

Read chapter 8.

DAY SIX

STEP ONE

Morning stretch, morning wake-up warm-ups, plus exercises for three special-attention spots, breakfast, shower or bath.

STEP TWO

Give yourself a complete monthly facial as outlined in chapter 2. Apply daily makeup.

Note: Don't forget your mineral or spring water.

STEP THREE

Take some form of physical activity such as a long walk (at least a mile), bicycling, tennis, swimming, horseback-riding, bowling, skating—whatever pleases you, but you must do *something*.

Lunch

one 8-ounce glass of Fruit Malted

P.M.

STEP ONE

    Begin alterations of the clothes you have selected for refashioning, or, if you are having someone else do the work, have your dressmaker come for fittings. (Some dry cleaners do alterations; you might want to check yours out if you do not know a dressmaker.)

DAY SEVEN

STEP ONE

Morning stretch, morning wake-up warm-ups, plus exercises for three special-attention spots, breakfast, shower or bath, daily skin-care routine, daily makeup.

STEP TWO

Go for your hair appointment. *Talk* to the hairdresser before he or she ever lays a hand on you. Given the basic style *you* have chosen, given the particular characteristics of *your* hair—fine, thick, wavy, straight, holds a curl or not, etc.—and given *your* particular life-style—work every day, swim a lot, many dress-up occasions, etc.—discuss how the style should be adapted to suit your individual needs. This is the only way to avoid looking wonderful when you leave the salon and then hating both your hairdresser and yourself after you get home and have to begin dealing with your new style by yourself on a day-to-day basis.

Lunch

one 8-ounce glass of Fruit Malted

15

P.M.

STEP ONE

Read chapter 9.

STEP TWO

Browse through a large magazine store and select a new magazine you have never read before with the idea that if you like it,you will subscribe to it. Don't get something that will look impressive on your coffee table. Get a magazine that interests *you*.

STEP THREE

Browse through a bookstore and buy one nonfiction book (hardcover or paperback) on a subject that seems interesting to you, on either an entirely new subject or on a subject in which you have previously been interested but have never had the time to explore.

Buy one other book in the self-help category—like one of those commonsense "How to Control Your Time and Life" books or "How Not to Feel Guilty," "How to Succeed," etc. (No health or beauty books; this step is for the inside.)

STEP FOUR

Read the magazine you have purchased. If you do like it, take out a year's subscription; if not, keep purchasing new magazines, one at a time, until you find one that does interest you and then take out the subscription.

STEP FIVE

Work on clothes alterations if necessary.

DAY EIGHT

STEP ONE

Morning stretch, morning wake-up warm-ups, plus exercises for three special-attention spots, breakfast, shower or bath, daily skin-care routine, daily makeup.

STEP TWO

Go shopping for:
1. fresh flowers for your bathroom
2. a new color of nail polish
3. a *new* perfume. After trying a *few*—any more than a few and your olfactory powers will fail you—select one new scent and buy the smallest bottle of cologne or toilet water or bath oil (the scent lasts longer) available, whichever is least expensive. You are still experimenting at this point, so it would be a waste of money to invest in an expensive perfume only to find that after wearing it for a week, you dislike it. Apply the new fragrance every day after your shower.

STEP THREE

Call a friend and make plans to see him/her for lunch—*at a restaurant* —on the eleventh day. (If you plan on having your hair professionally done for special occasions, call your hairdresser and make an appointment for the morning of the eleventh day.)

Lunch

one 8-ounce glass of Fruit Malted

Note: Don't forget your mineral or spring water.

P.M.

STEP ONE

Read your new self-improvement book. Read the entire book at one leisurely sitting, sipping on mineral water, eating a piece of fresh fruit and taking small breaks only if necessary.

Note down in "Work Sheets" three—and only three—things you will work on to improve yourself based on what you have learned from the book you have just read.

DAY NINE

STEP ONE

Morning stretch, morning wake-up warm-ups, plus exercises for three special-attention spots, breakfast, shower or bath, daily skin-care routine, daily makeup.

STEP TWO

Read chapter 10 and give yourself a manicure and a pedicure according to instructions.

STEP THREE

Go to your local high school adult-education department or your local "Y" or college extension department and find out what courses are available day and/or evening for adults. Select a course on a subject that interests you and enroll for next semester's class. You must enroll in something.

Lunch

one 8-ounce glass of Fruit Malted

19

P.M.

STEP ONE

Read chapter 11 on life-styles.

Do whatever you want all afternoon or evening. This doesn't mean do *nothing*. It takes thought and consideration of priorities to *decide* what you would like to do (which is the purpose of this time assignment). What do *you* really *want* to do? Make a list of pleasurable activities. Next, put them in order of preference. Then, do number one on the list —or the first one on the list that you can realistically do today—and set about to alter your life-style in such a way that you will be able to do all of the others on the list *on some level* as soon as possible.

DAY TEN

STEP ONE

Morning stretch, morning wake-up warm-ups, plus exercises for three special-attention spots, breakfast.

STEP TWO

Give yourself a "body" facial as outlined in chapter 2.

STEP THREE

Give yourself a "face" facial as outlined in chapter 2. (This can be done at the same time as the "body" facial, your beauty mask drying during the time spent on your body.)

STEP FOUR

Apply makeup as usual.

Lunch

one 8-ounce glass of Fruit Malted

21

P.M.

STEP ONE

Finish altering any clothes that still need it and examine your wardrobe for the last time (for now) to be sure that each and every item in it expresses the individual style that you have determined from your scrapbook. It may be a small wardrobe by now, but it is *yours*.

This is important! Even if your wardrobe is not yet quite right and even if you have made some mistakes in your choices or decisions, it is still better than it was, and it is still better than letting those decisions and choices be made by someone else. If you keep your scrapbook going and keep an interested eye on the subject, you will eventually add, subtract and alter with ease until you have achieved the right overall look for yourself. This is the *only* way to achieve an individual look. Unfortunately, there are no shortcuts to this end.

STEP TWO

Decide which fashion magazine would be best for you to subscribe to on a regular basis—consider your own style and your life-style. This will aid you in making your scrapbook a way of life. Take out a year's subscription to that magazine. (Be realistic. If you are over thirty-five, don't subscribe to *Seventeen*.)

STEP THREE

Begin the new nonfiction book you have purchased on your newly chosen subject.

DAY ELEVEN

OR *DAY ONE*
OF THE REST OF YOUR LIFE

Don't stop doing the things you've learned! It should be a way of life by now. If you get lazy, I assure you that you will gain back those ten years sooner than you imagine.

STEP ONE

Have your hair done professionally or do it fresh yourself.

STEP TWO

Meet your friend for lunch at the restaurant.

STEP THREE

Drop in on the man in your life (even if it's your husband) at his place of work, if that is permissible, and ask him "spur of the moment" (!!!) to take you out to dinner. Or go to a museum or browse through a store by yourself and plan to see a friend for dinner. This is "see people" day so that *you* can be seen.

STEP FOUR

Think "up," move "forward." These watchwords are reminders from me. "Up" in what manner, "forward" to where . . . it's up to you.

23

1

PUTTING AWAY OUR PLASTIC IDOLS

Cover girls, TV personalities and movie stars have lines around their eyes, get pimples and have to watch their weight.

You wouldn't think it would be necessary to point out such obvious truths, but in our increasingly bright and shiny, often "plastic" society, this seems to be the case. As a former actress and model, I can assure you from firsthand viewing and personal experience that what I tell you is true. And as a present speaker to women's groups the country over, I have assured myself that these truths need to be said.

Saddest of all, it isn't just women who seem (often secretly) to believe that certain people in our society are chosen for eternal youth and beauty; there are plenty of men who cherish this mistaken belief as well. Sometimes they relate the syndrome to themselves; but more often they relate it to women—especially *their* woman.

And now the truth about cover girls, film stars and public figures, as it pertains to our subjects of age and beauty:

The years are numbered for models in general as well as for those who appear regularly on the covers and within the pages of fashion magazines. All models know this. Most of their careers, as fashion models, are over somewhere between the ages of thirty and thirty-five. Many models move over to other types of print (magazine) modeling, where they can portray housewives or business executives or other mature women. Others go on, if they are actresses as well, to concentrate on television commercials; some become agents for modeling or casting agencies; others migrate to television or the movies—what they do afterward isn't important here. The important thing for you to realize is that most of those whom you see currently in magazines are actually young in years.

Even so, they are not, in person, what you see on the pages of your favorite magazine. Some have freckles or moles on their faces or bodies. Some have birth marks or scars (after all, they *are* people). Certainly most of them have, at one time or another, pimples in one place or another. Many of them have more lines around their eyes at any given age than the average, nonmodeling woman! One of the reasons for this is that many models begin their careers while still in their teens. Hence, they smile much, much more than the average person because smiling is part of their work. They also spend more time than is normal smiling into the sun, or squinting while waiting for the next shot; and when not out-of-doors, they are smiling into hot, drying lights.

During a photographic session, models may be twisted, turned, pinned and draped to camouflage any bodily imperfections they may have in order to achieve the "natural," "uncontrived" look. Wind machines are used extensively to create "natural," attractive effects. There was a story floating around in the fashion world a couple of years ago when America's latest Hollywood sex symbol posed for a bathing suit spread in one of the leading fashion magazines. It seems this actress was the athletic type and carried several small scars on her legs that were found to be unacceptable for the spread (because they made her human?). When the magazine appeared, this young woman was draped in some manner from the waist down in every, single shot—a shawl tied at the waist with only one lovely leg protruding, a towel flowing (thanks to a wind machine) over one leg. The message here is that, via the illusion-creating techniques available to photography, natural or accidental imperfections can be camouflaged out of existence. The angle of lighting alone can create shadows to flatter or fade or camouflage for a purpose.

Remember, too, that any single photographic session may result in a hundred or more pictures. One is chosen, or two, or six, but the point is that you, too, could find a few extraordinary pictures of yourself after a session with a professional photographer—first having your makeup, your hair and your clothing professionally designed—with dozens and dozens of photos from which to choose.

Aside from the above realities, photos that actually appear in magazines have been extensively retouched in all but the rarest instances. This is done by professionals who use a brush and watercolors or an instrument called an air brush or, in most cosmetic ads, bleaching and dyeing from a dye transfer of the original transparency. Lines around the eyes disappear completely or to any softened extent desired; moles and freckles vanish; shadows of underarm hair roots blend into the skin; lighting shadows falling at unattractive angles are cleared away; a towel or clothing that falls or drapes ungracefully is softened to create a trimmer curve. Countless other realities can be eliminated, or illusions created, through the skillful use of retouching. One of the sure signs, by the way, to enable you to detect retouching in any photo is that many of them carry a "too-perfect" look. If you believe the real girl really looks that way, you are the only one you are fooling.

I would like to stress here that I am not trying to downgrade or take away any of the glamour of the modeling profession. Many models are lovely and beautiful in person. It is not a sin to retouch. What I am trying to make clear is that the women you see on the covers of magazines are people too, just as you are, subject to the whole range of human imperfections and problems. If a *model* gains five pounds, she could lose a job! Do not feel that your looks are in any way inferior just because you don't seem to measure up to the one-in-a-hundred shot of the retouched girl who is still under thirty whom you find smiling out at you from the pages of any particular magazine.

In films, as well, numberless techniques are utilized to create the exact image desired. Lighting angles can make or break the features of an actress's face. Everyone has heard the statement "The camera 'loves' her." Some people are more photogenic than others. Film makeup is crucial—don't forget, it is applied by professionals. Much attention is paid to hair color, styles, etc. Costumes are designed specifically, again by professionals, for each individual actress in order to accent her assets and detract from her defects.

And don't forget that most actors and actresses as well as many public figures (at least the ones you are jealous of) spend much of their own time and money and *effort* on their faces and physiques. They spend weeks at spas each year to keep in shape; they exercise daily (often two hours or more) to maintain their physical condition; they get regular, professionals facials, wear designer clothes and have cosmetic surgery. There is nothing wrong with any of this—part of their profession depends upon their appearance. Just remember that if you, too, spent this much time and money on your outward appearance, you would look as good as they do.

The only reason I offer this chapter in this book at all is because I have sadly learned in my travels and by meeting women from one end of the country to the other that many people do not realize just what goes into the making of magazines and movies to create the illusions you wish were reality—especially on your own body and face. Public figures have private, *real* lives too. You just don't see them.

You also don't see, in person, the beneficiaries of professional make-overs a week after their make-over. Remember when viewing photographs in books or magazines of average women who have undergone a make-over by one professional or another that you are viewing just that— a photograph. The subject's hair, makeup and clothing were created by professionals for that one session with a professional photographer; and the "before" pictures are usually too bad to be true, the women made to look so terrible (in many cases unbelievably so), that *anything* would be an improvement. This is not to imply that the lessons learned and new styles adopted by any woman who has chosen to be made over are not worthwhile, but do not be led to the false conclusion that any such woman looks that astoundingly transformed when she begins to create the new look for herself with her own untrained hands. The secret is not to be made over by someone else, but to learn to create your best look yourself; the results are much more dependable that way.

And there are, happily, many things you can do to improve your own appearance dramatically. Following the advice in this book on a regular basis, after your ten-day program is over, is one of them. Keeping your weight down and exercising regularly to keep your muscles toned is another. Cosmetic surgery is available to you, too. As far as your *personal* appearance is concerned, as opposed to photographed or filmed illusionary appearances, you have as much available to you, given determination, time and/or money, as does any public figure you admire.

The decision is yours to make. But, for your own sake, do not be discouraged by what may seem to be the existence of a few, chosen people who appear to retain youth and beauty beyond your ability to do so. It simply isn't true. In the real world, nobody can eat her cake and keep her figure, too.

Since we're setting records straight, perhaps a word or two should be said here concerning the subject of age itself. You want to look younger. I want to help you; otherwise I would not have written this book. But you should not want, and I cannot help you obtain, an unrealistic goal. If you are five foot three, neither of us can make you five foot seven. If you have straight hair, neither of us can make it naturally curly. If you are forty, neither of us can turn you, in actual years, back to twenty-five. You are the only you you have.

One can change oneself, and can continue to improve—both inwardly and outwardly—on a regular basis. But pining for what once was is only a confession that one is not satisfied now. Pining for something that can never be is so unrealistic it only results in paralysis of motivation. Today's current cultural values, which focus with a tenacious fanaticism upon the desire for eternal youth, unfortunately do not help; in fact, they only encourage both men and women to yearn for impossible goals.

Current career requirements, which often require youth in years, can also be terribly demoralizing. Many over-forty people of both sexes face a depressingly difficult time making job changes or advancements because the emphasis is so often fixed on the young. Why, I cannot explain, because logic would indicate that a more mature person could offer more expertise. Nevertheless, even if these career hurdles are thrown up in front of you, you must not permit yourself to take them deeply to heart; they must never diminish *your* view of you (easier said than done, I realize, but worth remembering).

The current fashion emphasis remains focused on the kinky, "freaky," "costumey" looks of the young. This is all right, of course, for the young in years, because experimentation is part of growing up. They are still discovering and creating their identities. But you should have a good idea of yours by now. You should be dressing like *you*, not like your daughter. What are you promising her from adulthood if you keep emulating *her*? In today's fashion world, there exist choices enough for anyone of any age to express her own individuality.

If you have not yet found your individuality, that is where your efforts should be directed. In appearance as well as in attitude. Age, in actual years, is not really a factor of major focus to someone who *is* what she wants to be. If you are not what you wish to be, you can change. Now. Getting your outward appearance into shape can not only be an exciting adventure in its own right, but it can also be an enormous primer for inner motivation. If "younger" really means the fittest and most attractive and vibrant outward appearance you can achieve; if it means purposeful activity (different from nonstop distraction), inner growth, extra energy and optimistic anticipation of the future—you can acquire or maintain all of these qualities of youth at any chronological age.

So, welcome to the *real* world . . . and, just perhaps, the real you.

2

SOME SKIN SENSE

One of the most amazing aspects of today's beauty scene is the number of people who spend hundreds of dollars at the cosmetic counter on the word of a salesperson or the promise of a magazine ad, without ever knowing in their own minds what is really required for the care of their skin or, for that matter, what is required for the care of *any* skin by the physical nature of human skin itself. The list of ingredients on the back of the package does you absolutely no good if you don't know what each ingredient is contributing (or not contributing) toward the daily health of your own skin.

So while we're talking straight, let's get rid of some more myths. Your skin will never look like the retouched skin of the girl in the magazine ad or the girl—selected especially for her perfect skin out of hundreds who applied—in the TV commercial. It will always look like *your* skin because it *is* your skin. However, it certainly can—and should—look like the loveliest, clearest, youngest skin *you* can have.

Note: If you are really the impatient, "I've got to see results immediately"–type person, you can go to chapter 5 on makeup and read and learn the immediate result makeup can offer first. However, be advised that unless you, tomorrow, begin caring for your skin properly—not just making it up skilfully —you will never, in the long run, achieve the youthful look you want.

Understanding Your Skin

Most of us don't think of the skin as an organ. But it is; it is, in fact, the largest organ of our entire body. The surface covers about nineteen square feet, weighs an average of seven pounds, and varies in thickness from one-thirty-second to one-eighth of an inch. This organ, which is 98 percent protein, is not only large but complex as well. One square inch of skin contains approximately three yards of blood vessels, three hundred sweat glands, twelve yards of nerves, six hundred nerve endings, thirty hairs, and forty-five oil glands. All that is worth caring for.

A healthy, hence beautiful, skin is soft to the touch, yet firm, because of an inherent elasticity. It is moist, with a definite acid balance. In texture, good skin is smooth and fine-grained. In color, it is uniform and glows with life.

Most of the skin's basic attributes—color, texture, aging tendencies—are inherited. Luckily, we live in an age in which science can tell us what to do with our inherited package to correct nature's mistakes. Science's vital information, however, must be evaluated in terms of our own individual skins. In order to do that, it is first necessary to understand something, in principle, about this marvelous organ.

Everyone's skin is made up of two main layers. The outermost layer, the one that protects everything underneath, is called the *epidermis*. Besides its main function as protector of all the other organs, it also contains a rich nerve supply. This nerve network responds to touch, pain and pressure, as well as to heat and cold, both sending sensory messages to the brain and acting as a thermostat reporting the temperature outside so that the system can adjust its internal controls to keep you comfortable.

The epidermis itself has several layers, but it will serve our purpose here to examine only the bottom layer, technically termed the *basal* layer. It is the function of the cells of this layer to continually renew the life of your skin. They divide, and while the newly created cells carry on the life processes, the previously existing cells are progressively carried to the surface of the skin. Because they cannot survive exposure to air and water, they grow old there and eventually die. Then they are gradually shed. It is because of this very efficient system of sloughing off the old, dead skin only to reveal new, fresh skin that we are able to maintain a soft, young-looking skin. A side benefit of this proces is the skin's built-in ability to eradicate superficial scars in this manner.

Immediately beneath the epidermis—which literally means "upon the dermis"—is situated, logically enough, the *dermis*. This second layer is sometimes referred to as the "true skin." It is made up of a protein fiber that acounts for most of the skin's elasticity. Time alone weakens the fiber, and so, with age, the elasticity is diminished, the skin becomes looser and thinner and wrinkles begin to appear.

The dermis extends deeper into a kind of cushion of fatty, subcutaneous tissue that has the very special function of feeding the skin and rendering it free of toxins and waste materials.

Although most of us may not be aware of these layers beneath the surface of the skin, we are all aware of the oil glands situated at the base of each hair on our body—aware of them, usually, because they put out too much or too little oil. It is these *sebaceous* glands, as they are technically called, that provide the protective oil balance, called *sebum*, that appears on the surface of the skin. You've undoubtedly been aware of visible oil on your own or someone else's forehead. Sebum tends to be more apparent in that area because the center of the forehead (along with the scalp, nose and chin) contains more sebaceous glands than any other area of the entire body. If you blot the oil off, it will only replace itself within a short time. This process is the skin's automatic method of protecting itself against the outside elements.

(Many women have complexion problems around menstruation time. This is because there is a rise in the activity of the sebaceous glands on or about the twelfth to fifteenth day of the menstrual cycle, and then this rather high level is maintained until the onset of menstruation. If you experience breakouts on your face periodically each month, this is probably the reason.)

The entire skin organ has as its special duty the eliminative functions of the body. It virtually breathes for the body through the pores in very much the same manner as the lungs do, but, of course, on a much smaller scale. Oxygen is taken in and carbon dioxide is discharged. Water, too, is eliminated—approximately a pint of it on an average day (now you see the need for moisturizing creams and the need to drink plenty of water each day). The skin also rids the body of any toxins that may be harmful.

I've already mentioned the oils that come to the surface for natural elimination by the skin. Some of them, of course, don't always succeed in rising through the surface and become trapped beneath it. If they can't be secreted, the skin then has the ability to oxidize them. This forces them out in the form of a blemish.

Besides the capacity to eliminate substances from the system, the skin is also able to do the reverse. It has a limited ability to absorb. "Limited" because if it could take things in as readily as it lets them out, we would all be in serious peril. The skin seems to have the very good discriminative ability to absorb, predominately via the hair follicles and sebaceous glands, those things that aid the body—like natural oils from a good cream—and at the same time refuse admission to poisons and toxins in the air.

One of the precautions the skin takes to keep out harmful bacteria and other infection is to cloak itself with an *acid mantle*. This function is actually a matter of maintaining the proper acid-alkaline balance, but for good health, it must lean toward the acid, so this balance has been termed an "acid mantle." This is the *pH factor*, a term with which you are all, undoubtedly, familiar. The pH is a measurement of the acidity or alkalinity of any substance.

You can buy nitrazine paper to test for pH at the drugstore. It's yellow and comes in a little dispenser. If you dip it into any cosmetic, bath oil, or soap, it turns color. There is a color scale right on the package ranging from pH 4.5 to pH 7.5. Anything that registers 7 or below is acidic. Anything that registers above 7 is alkaline.

The acid mantle or balance of the skin ranges between 4.2 and 4.6; so the most compatible products to use on your face would be those that fall within that range. Anything above a pH-7 level, if used at all, should be followed by a skin freshener to replace the skin's normal acidity. This is especially true for a physically aging face. As the skin grows older, it loses its own ability to restore the natural acid balance that every skin requires.

Washing your face with soap and water will be discussed later, but it's timely to note here that, while I have tested dozens of soaps with nitrazine paper, I have found only a few with the same acidity level as the skin. Most of them are alkaline, which actually promotes dryness. The skin ages soon enough all by itself, without any additional assistance from cleansers and beauty aids that "aid" you only to premature lines and wrinkles.

After about the age of thirty, the skin just naturally becomes drier. This is the age when most women will begin to see lines near the eyes and mouth. But not you (now lucky) women with the same oily skin that has plagued you from adolescence. Since your sebaceous glands are naturally overactive, they'll keep you in soft, dewy skin years longer than your dry-skinned sisters who now need to stimulate and replenish their oil wells with primers from a bottle.

Caring for Your Skin

Beautiful skin, no matter what the type, demands constant care to resist the aging process. And the earlier you begin, the better. You'll notice the loss of elasticity first in your neck. This is a warning signal, and the face is next. Massaging properly with moisturizing creams will help tone the underlying muscles of the face and slow down the inevitable. And that's precisely what we're attempting to accomplish with all skins. You cannot *stop* the process of aging, but you surely can slow it down. Simple things, like making sure the water in your home is "soft" (by purchasing a water softener if necessary) and using a humidifier in winter (when the artificial heat in your home or office is robbing your skin of its natural moisture) will do their share in retarding the aging process. But the most important method of maintaining a healthy, young skin is to cleanse, tone, moisturize and care for it every day of your life.

Caring for the skin externally is not, however, all that the skin requires to stay young and beautiful.

What goes *onto* your body surely is important, but never underestimate the value of what goes *into* your body as well.

A nutritious, well-balanced diet is crucial. A good share of protein— lean meats, fish, poultry and eggs— plus fruits, vegetables, grains, dairy products and adequate quantities of water all help to keep you strong, healthy and functioning efficiently on the inside. If your internal organs are malfunctioning, the resulting toxins can spread to the bloodstream, where they will be transported to the skin for elimination. This procedure is normal and proper, but the frequency of such a demand on the skin is a factor determining its own health. It is possible literally to overwork the skin organ. Its elasticity, texture and color can all be adversely affected by improper nutrition.

If what goes into your body is critical, *how much* is important, too. If the proportion is not sufficient, it could result in a vitamin deficiency. There is impressive evidence that a lack of vitamins—especially A (green and yellow vegetables), D (milk) and B (liver)—directly affects the health of the skin. These nutrients can be supplemented with foods such as cod liver oil (vitamins A and D) or brewer's yeast (vitamin B) or with vitamin pills, but every effort should be made to ensure the skin the benefit of these vitamins. If vitamin C (the infection-fighting vitamin) is insufficient in the diet, the skin may also mirror the loss.

My purpose here is not to offer concrete advice on nutrition but merely to bring the subject of diet to your general attention.

A parallel consideration that also has an effect for good or ill on the skin is exercise (discussed in some detail in chapters 4 and 8). The fitness of the rest of your body is reflected in the appearance of your facial skin. Sedentary bodies usually result in dull skin. Exercise stimulates all internal organs to function smoothly; it distributes the nutrients just discussed; it tones the muscles and it eradicates fatigue and stress. It gets that wonderful machine that is your body *moving*. It encourages life.

As can be seen, then, it is necessary to attend to your whole package, not just the wrapping. Care for the health of your whole body . . . outside *and* inside. Your skin will show the results.

Before I leave the general care of the skin, the issue of suntanning should be explored. Much has been written on this subject, and too much, I fear, has had an hysterical quality to it. Moderate suntanning is not going to give you skin cancer in ten minutes. The sun can be beneficial to your skin as well as harmful. Common sense must be used, that's all.

The sun causes the skin to produce vitamin D, which is necessary for health. It stimulates the skin to produce a honey-brown glow that usually creates a youthful look.

The sun also has a drying effect on the skin. In cases of oily or troubled skins, this can be helpful. The sun gives life, warmth and light.

It's only our misuse of the sun that can bring us harm. Reasonable behavior is in order. Even cautious behavior. Because as well as causing a lovely, lush tan, given enough time the sun can also cause a very painful and not at all lovely burn. And even a moderate sunburn is potentially harmful to the normal function of skin cells. Inflammation caused by a burn can actually damage the cells.

But with a little common sense, those very same cells will work for you instead of against you. Small doses of sunlight will stimulate them to increase a brown pigment called *melanin*. The melanin protects your skin against larger doses of sun, and so the cycle is established in your favor. The brown pigment is the tan we're all after.

Caution, not panic, is desirable too against the drying attributes of the sun. Even if you tan easily and need no protection against the burning potential of the sun, you do need protection against its dehydrating potential.

Fortunately, neither burning nor drying by the sun is a major problem. Protection against both is achieved simply and inexpensively by the application of an appropriate sunscreen.

Note: Most sunscreens do not prevent the sun's rays from reaching the skin, so exposure must be limited. What a good sunscreen does do is absorb a certain percentage of the ultraviolet rays, thus reducing the intensity of the sun's powers. This gives your skin a chance to build up its own protection, which is the tan you wanted in the first place.

Certain natural oils can be used as sunscreens, since they, too, absorb the ultraviolet rays. Natural sesame oil, for example, absorbs 39 percent of these rays and therefore makes an excellent, lubricating suntan oil. If you purchase ready-made, commercial lotions, the inclusion of PABA (para-aminobenzoic acid) in the ingredients will give you added protection.

If a lubricant or sunscreen is *not* used, then the results truly will be a dry, prematurely aged skin. But with the proper care, I can find no facts to substantiate claims that moderate exposure to the sun is a danger to any normally functioning skin.

It should be mentioned here, too, that the facts of the matter also do not support the current, alarmist assertions that skin cancer is a threat to average sunbathers. Skin cancer is an occupational hazard of both farmers and sailors, it is true. And it can be caused by the sun. That is also true. But people working in either of these fields are exposed all day, every day, for years on end to the drying effects of the sun. Their skin is seldom if ever protected by even a lubricant, let alone a sunscreen. And with all of this abuse, cases of skin cancer are still rare. I really do not think it looms as a major danger for any normal, reasonable sunbather.

If you wish to bask in the sun, I would say to have fun doing it. Just don't let it burn you, and don't go after a deep tan.

How to Find Your Own Skin Type

Before you learn how to care for your skin, you must learn just what type of skin you have. Cosmeticians divide skin types into three main categories: normal, oily and dry. It is also possible to have a combination of any of these three groups on the same face. For example, you might have an oily "T" zone (forehead, nose and chin) with the rest of the facial skin dry. Any combination you may have is aptly labeled a *combination* skin. It's a bit of trouble, practically speaking, because you must care for each zone differently, thereby making it necessary to use a few more beauty aids. The great majority of women *do* have combination skins, however, so if you do, you are not alone.

If you buy commercial cleansers and creams, you cannot possibly do it intelligently without knowing your own skin type. (Remember, if you use ready-made cosmetics, that the labeled ingredients—if you can decipher their technical names—are listed on the package in declining order according to their respective amounts in the product. If you see "water" listed first, that means there is more water in the product than any other ingredient, and so on down the line.) If you decide to make your own products, you need to know your type in order to select appropriate recipes.

The simplest way to determine your skin type, and also the most enjoyable, is to go to a salon and have an analysis and a facial. This is a real treat and can prove to be continually beneficial even after you start your at-home routine. Most salons suggest that you come in once every month or six weeks for a professional facial and then maintain a regular skin-care program at home between visits. At the salon, they'll settle you into a reclining lounge, tuck you in with a pretty coverlet and then proceed to cleanse and pamper your face, neck and shoulders for nearly an hour. Most salons will try to sell you their products after the facial, so forewarned is forearmed; you may or may not buy. (Although I think the analysis from a professional is a valid method of determining your skin type, I do not recommend the computer analyses offered by some cosmetic companies. I have checked out several, and not one came up with my exact skin type. You must understand that the questions asked are not specific enough or complete enough or individual enough to be able to take into account your own skin characteristics. Especially if you have combination skin, as most of us do, you are likely to come away with an incorrect or misleading analysis, which would then throw your whole skin-care program off the track. At best, computers can give you a general idea of your skin type.)

You do not need, however, even a professional, salon analysis to determine your own skin type. So, if there's no salon in your town, or if you don't want to spend the money, or if you're just not interested, you can very easily analyze your own skin. Even if you have your skin professionally analyzed, I would suggest you confirm the diagnosis yourself; professionals are not infallible.

First, get hold of a magnifying mirror if you can. It's not absolutely necessary, but if you have one handy it will make the job easier. Now look carefully (and honestly) at your face. The following guide will help you make a correct analysis.

NORMAL SKIN

This is the rarest type of all. I never have been able to understand why it's called "normal" skin. It's the kind of skin we're all trying to achieve. If you find it's your type, consider yourself chosen and be certain to take care of it to keep it that way. Normal skin is young, fresh, firm, moist, fine-grained, supple skin with a smooth texture. It is free from blemishes.

You must keep an eye on this type of skin because eventually, as you get older, you will probably end up with dry skin. So watch carefully for dryness, and when it arrives, switch to a dry-skin-care routine. The first signs will be a taut feeling to your face when the weather turns cold and a general sensitivity to the elements. Also, if you wash with most soaps (which will probably speed you toward those dry days), you'll experience a tight feeling afterward.

DRY OR DEHYDRATED SKIN

Dry skin is a sign of sluggish or underactive oil glands and/or the inability of your skin to produce or retain enough water moisture. You will have a tendency toward early lines and wrinkles.

Other clues to this skin type are the presence of small pore openings and fine lines on a thin skin. With your fingertips, push the skin upward; if you see the formation of tiny lines, that's a pretty sure sign. If you burn or peel easily in the sun and chap easily in the wind and cold, and if you get a tight feeling in cold weather or after a soap and water wash, you can be assured of your diagnosis. If your skin occasionally appears or feels parched and has a tendency to flake, it is seriously dry.

Dry skin needs not only constant vigilance but also protection against the elements. You'll need the benefits of a moisturizing cream at all times, but especially in winter when the artificial heat in your home or office results in a loss of humidity in the air, hence a loss of moisture from your skin. Be sure to drink several glasses of water each day, be sure to use only soft water to wash your skin (if your water is hard, it is well worth the investment to buy a water softener) and be sure to keep a humidifier going at all times in winter.

A deep tan is not for you, whether from the beach or the ski slopes.

Be sure to smooth on a good sunscreen with an oil base. Your skin can be stunning because it is so delicate, but you will have to pamper it a bit more than other types.

OILY SKIN

If you have trouble with any degree or kind of acne condition during adolescence, you probably still have oily skin at present. Not always, of course, because nerves, diet, hormonal imbalance and many other factors play a significant role in creating skin problems. So look for other signs to support your suspicion. If your skin has an oily appearance on the surface, this may be evidence of a deeper oily condition. If your skin is susceptible to blackheads and/or small bumps beneath the surface, you are likely to fall into this category. Enlarged pores are another phenomenon to check for. Most women know if they have oily skin.

If you do, it's a type to be relentlessly cared for. And not with tender, loving care, but with firm, no-nonsense discipline. Remember, however, that your skin will continue getting lovelier each year as your extra oil output moistens it to a beautiful "normal" condition. Watch for indications that your overactive oil wells are slowing down, and switch skin-care regimes accordingly.

When you apply skin-care products to this skin type, you must exercise caution in one respect; caring for an oily skin does not mean robbing it of *all* of its oils. If you strip away all of these natural moisturizers, your skin will not be able to maintain the necessary balance of oils and water that it properly needs. What you must do is keep the face free of *excess* oiliness; if you kept your skin absolutely dry of oils, you would soon experience the same early aging tendencies a person with dry skin does.

COMBINATION SKIN

The most frequent kind of *combination* skin is part oily and part normal or dry. You can readily see the excess oil on the forehead and possibly the nose area. Perhaps it's not so discernible on the chin, but if you have a blemish problem, however sporadic, in that zone, the chin is probably oily, too. Check for enlarged pores and tiny blackheads or whiteheads hiding under the surface of the skin, which give it a grainy appearance. The cheeks, including the jawline and the outer edges of the forehead, will most likely be dry or normal. Scrutinize all sections of your face carefully to determine the type of each.

Combination skin requires slightly more effort than the other types, but it's not formidable. You must simply treat and care for each zone separately: oily lotions and masks for the areas needing them and dry or normal treatments for the rest.

AGING SKIN

It is never too late to improve your appearance by acquiring a good skin-care program. Even if you are entering or well into your later years, there is still a great deal you can do, not only to restore a more youthful look but also to retard outward appearances of the inevitable aging process. As long as any damage to the skin is confined to the outer layer, most signs of neglect or aging can be substantially improved.

If any damage has occurred to the dermis, or inner layer, there is really little if anything that can be accomplished by external beauty care. Since the dermis cannot regenerate itself as the outer layer can, any structural damage is usually permanent. Whether the damage has occurred from illness, accident or neglect, the signs will often begin to show with age, because, as we have seen, it is the dermis that determines the tone or elasticity of the skin. When it loses resilience, the supporting tissue underneath the dermis lose their strength and the whole face begins to sag. Structural collapse, serious wrinkle problems and scars caused by damage to the dermis are the province of the medical profession. If these are your problems and you wish to correct them, you should consult a reputable cosmetic surgeon.

However, if the damage has occurred only to the epidermis, or outer layer, the outlook for dramatic improvement is bright indeed. One of the correctable problems of aging skin is the rough or pasty appearance that results when it loses its ability to shed the dead skin cells on the surface, leaving them there to build up. That's why it's crucial, once or twice a week, to use a cleansing cream that contains mildly abrasive granules. These little "beauty grains," as we might call them, scrub the dead layer of skin off the surface and leave your face with a younger look immediately (see "Anti-age Skin Routines" at the end of this chapter).

Another problem common with aging skin is chronic dryness. There are several reasons for this. One is simply the decreased activity of the sebaceous glands—they are simply running out of oil. Another is that, with age, the skin loses its ability to restore the acid balance to the skin if it is altered for any reason; for example, washing with an alkaline soap. Thus a skin freshener is an absolute necessity for aging skin; it replaces the protective acid mantle usually washed away in cleansing. Lastly, the outer cells become less able to hold water, which is, of course, the real moisturizer, and so the skin begins to take on a parched look. The resulting dryness makes an old skin look older, hence the imperative need for a good moisturizing program. Be sure, too, to use only soft water for washing, use a humidifier in the winter and drink plenty of water every day.

The final insult to aging skin can be a pigment increase in the outer layer. This wouldn't really matter if it increased evenly, but it tends to do so in a "here and there" pattern that often causes an unattractive, splotchy look. This phenomenon is sometimes referred to as "liver spots," but I couldn't tell you why, since it has nothing whatsoever to do with the liver.

Obviously, because of these special attributes of aging skin, special care must be given to it. But even if all of your problems seem a little grim, and even if your own face in the mirror shows its age, do not be in the slightest discouraged. With special care, skin can be dewy and youthful—belying its age—within a very short time.

Daily Skin-Care Regimes for All Types of Skin

Each skin type demands a routine specifically designed to meet its individual needs, which you will find immediately following, but the general program is the same for all. Every type requires thorough cleansing and moisturizing or protection. In the morning and again before you retire (never go to bed wearing makeup!), every skin needs cleansing with a cream or oil in order to remove makeup, unclog pores of dirt and grime and let the skin breathe in order to fulfill its role as an eliminative organ.

If you wish to use a soap and water wash, that would come next. Oily skins can actually benefit from a soap wash because, since most soaps are alkaline, they act to dry the skin. Those with dry skin wishing to wash with soap and water should select only superfatted soaps and check the pH factor with nitrazine paper to be sure it is acidic. Those with aging skin would do best to stay away from soap and water altogether.

An all-important skin freshener follows to restore the pH factor and tone and freshen the skin, as well as to finish the cleaning process. If you don't believe that skin fresheners are crucial to your skin care, please experiment with the following test: Clean your face the usual way until you are certain that it is clean. Next, in a bottle, mix 1 ounce of witch hazel with 1 tablespoon of alcohol, if your skin is dry, or 2 tablespoons of alcohol if your skin is oily, plus 1 tablespoon of fresh, strained grapefruit juice or brandy. Shake well. Now, apply your home-made skin freshener to a cotton ball and, remembering that you are wiping dirt *off* your face, not wiping the freshener *on*, clean your face completely with upward and outward strokes. The amount of dirt you see on the cotton is the amount of dirt you walk around with on your face every day if you do not use a skin freshener.

After the skin freshener comes eye cream to soften and diminish the appearance of lines and wrinkles around the eye area. Lastly comes the application of a moisturizing or protection cream, which serves to soften and lubricate the skin as well as to help to maintain its vital oil and water balance. By forming a light film over the surface of the skin, a good cream or oil helps in the retention of water beneath the surface, thus maintaining the skin's natural moisture. In addition, this cream protects the skin under makeup and against the elements.

You may ask, "Is that all?"—and rightly so. With all the specialty products on the market, it would surely be reasonable to wonder about any possible added value of ultrarich night creams, under-makeup moisturizers, etc. In my judgment, anything more than the previously mentioned beauty aids is superfluous for daily skin care. A good cream moisturizes, softens and protects your skin at any hour, day or night. I can find no physiological reason to have separate beauty aids for morning, for under makeup or for before bed.

As you can see, the procedures are, in principle, the same for all skin types. More specific and refined routines are outlined at the end of this chapter. However, the products used should be drastically different, since each skin type needs help in its own special way. Also, reexamine your skin anew from time to time; it changes from season to season and from year to year.

THE DIFFERENCES AMONG CREAMS

The most important principle affecting moisturizing or protection creams centers on the subject of oils. Most all creams, whether you make them at home or buy them in a store, are simply a combination of waxes, oils and water. What makes the difference is the fact that mineral-oil-based creams will not penetrate the skin and natural and animal-oil-based creams will, to some extent. When you apply most commercial products to the skin and see them "penetrate," it is usually only the water in the cream evaporating, merely giving you the *sense* of penetration. If an oil is to truly penetrate, it takes a few minutes.

Obviously, if you have oily skin, you do not want any more oils to penetrate into the sebaceous glands. It would only aggravate your already aggravating condition. Therefore, creams that contain mineral oil would be best for you. They will soften and lubricate and protect your skin without providing additional oil.

A dry skin, conversely (and especially an *aging*, dry skin), can benefit from a cream containing oils that *will* penetrate the surface of the skin. Animal oils (lanolin, for example) and natural, cold-pressed vegetable oils (almond, sesame, olive) have the ability to penetrate, to some extent, the sebaceous glands and supplement the oil there, or even act as a primer to induce sluggish glands themselves to produce more oil. (If you want to see this work, apply a natural vegetable oil daily to an oily skin and watch it break out in blemishes within a few days because it can't handle the extra oil.) Mineral-oil-based creams are certainly better than nothing for a dry skin; they at least lubricate it, but they do not moisturize it. Therefore, in this book, I will consistently refer to "moisturizing" creams—meaning creams based in natural oils—for dry and aging skins, and "protection" creams—meaning creams based in mineral oils—for oily skins.

Weekly Beauty Masks for All Types of Skin

A weekly beauty mask can be applied for a variety of reasons, depending on your own individual needs and skin type. A mask can tighten your skin and minimize pore size, giving the overall appearance a fine-textured polish; it can bleach; it can penetrate and moisturize; it can act as a superficial or defoliating peeler to rid the face of accumulated dead skin cells. If the ingredients in the mask contain protein, it can even possibly repair superficially damaged skin. Whatever your specific purpose, however, there is one crucial function all masks should fulfill, and that is to cleanse the skin *internally*. It is this process that really brings youth back to any skin.

Internal cleansing is necessary for all adult skins of all types. A mask, by way of heat or a drying effect, stimulates circulation and draws blood to the surface of the skin, which oxygenates or feeds its underlying tissues. On the blood's return trip, it takes along with it any toxins or bacteria that may have been hiding just beneath the surface of the skin. It is this elimination of impurities beneath the outward appearance of your skin that encourages the surface to glow again with vibrancy and youth. Daily skin-care routines, no matter how thorough, cannot give you this all-important deep cleansing; that is why the regular application of a beauty mask seems to work such magic on a skin that has not previously benefited from the process. If you are faithful to a weekly or biweekly beauty mask, only then can your cleansing creams and skin fresheners and your moisturizers effectively maintain a fresh, dewy complexion on all the days in between. (When applying a beauty mask, be sure to cover the neck area as well.)

If, by chance, you experience a breakout problem following your first couple of beauty masks, do not be concerned. If your skin is unaccustomed to this deep-cleaning technique, it may utilize these introductory sessions to rid itself of buried impurities that have accumulated, unfortunately, over a rather long period of time.

Complete Daily, Weekly and Monthly
"Anti-age" Skin-Care Routines Individualized to Your Type

Once you get into the habit, it will require no more than ten minutes for your daily skin care no matter what your type, and the results will be well worth it. The important thing is to establish the habit. Morning and night. *Every* morning and *every* night. More often if you wish, but at least make it a policy to cleanse and moisturize your face thoroughly upon rising in the morning and before retiring at night.

Then add to that your weekly beauty mask and a monthly facial and

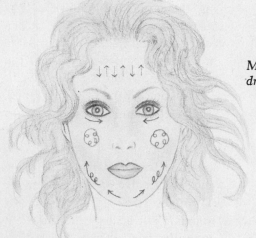

Massage techniques for normal, dry, combination and aging skins

you have the entire anti-age routine. If you would like to apply a superficial peeler or defoliating mask, do it in place of the beauty mask when you give yourself a complete facial.

Although, as we have already seen, the general guidelines are fundamentally the same for all skin types, there are some obvious and crucial differences. Because of that, individual beauty routines are listed separately under skin types. Find your type and you're on your way.

(Dry, normal, aging and combination skins note illustration for massaging technique used to apply moisturizing creams.)

ANTI-AGE ROUTINES FOR NORMAL SKIN

Morning Routine

1. Smooth cleansing cream over face. Massage well and remove with several tissues *or* rinse face with warm water and remove cream with wet, warm washcloth (clean washcloth daily).

2. This step is optional, but if you want to wash with soap and water, now is the time.

3. With short, firm strokes upward and outward, cleanse entire face with cotton balls or pads moistened with skin freshener. Use fresh cotton as needed until pad is free of dirt.

4. Apply moisturizing cream and massage deeply.

5. Apply eye cream.

6. Blot off any excess cream.

Midday Touchup

1. Keep "crinkle stick" (recipe in chapter 3) or a small pot of petroleum jelly in your bag, and when you repair your makeup during the day, pat the stick sparingly and gently over any wrinkled area (right over makeup) around the eyes, mouth, etc.

2. Blot off any grime with a tissue lightly moistened with warm water or skin freshener.

Evening Routine

1. Apply cleansing cream over entire face and throat. Gently but firmly remove makeup with several clean tissues.

2. Apply cleansing cream for a second time and remove as usual.

3. Optional wash with soap and water.

4. Remove any remaining dirt or makeup with skin freshener.

5. Apply moisturizing cream and massage face thoroughly.

6. Apply eye cream.

Weekly Routine

1. Cleanse face as usual with cleansing cream.
2. Optional wash with soap and water
3. Follow with skin freshener.
4. Steam face for ten minutes (recipe in chapter 3).
5. Apply beauty mask of your choice and leave on for amount of time specified in recipe or apply purchased product.
6. Remove mask and rinse face thoroughly. Pat dry.
7. Apply skin freshener.
8. Apply moisturizing cream. Massage deeply.
9. Apply eye cream.
10. Blot off excess cream.

Monthly Facial

1. Cleanse face as usual with cleansing cream.
2. Optional wash with soap and water.
3. Follow with skin freshener.
4. Apply moisturizing cream to face. Massage thoroughly.
5. Cover face with warm, wet washcloth and lie down to rest for five minutes.
6. Remove cream with skin freshener.
7. Steam face for five to ten minutes. Pat dry.
8. Apply a defoliating beauty mask. Place cotton pads soaked in rosewater or witch hazel over eyes.
9. Lie down and rest for specified time.
10. Remove mask and rinse face thoroughly. Pat dry.
11. Apply skin freshener.
12. Apply moisturizing cream. Massage deeply.
13. Apply eye cream.
14. Blot off excess cream.

ANTI-AGE ROUTINES FOR DRY SKIN

Morning Routine

1. Smooth cleansing cream over face. Massage well. Place very warm, wet washcloth over face two or three times. Remove cream with washcloth (clean washcloth daily).
2. This step is optional, but if you want to wash with soap and water, now is the time.
3. With short, firm strokes upward and outward, cleanse entire face

with cotton pads moistened in skin freshener. Use fresh cotton as needed and cleanse until pad is free of dirt.

4. Spray face lightly with mineral fater.
5. Apply moisturizing cream and massage deeply.
6. Apply eye cream.
7. Blot off excess cream.
8. Spray face lightly with mineral water and let dry naturally.

Midday Touchup

1. Keep "crinkle stick" (recipe in chapter 3) or small pot of petroleum jelly in your bag, and when you repair your makeup during the day, pat the stick sparingly and gently over any wrinkled area (right over makeup) around the eyes, mouth, etc.

Evening Routine

1. Apply cleansing cream over entire face. Gently but firmly remove makeup with several clean tissues or squares of cotton padding soaked in warm water.
2. Apply cleansing cream for a second time and remove as usual.
3. Optional wash with soap and water.
4. Remove any remaining dirt or makeup with skin freshener.
5. Spray face lightly with mineral water.
6. Apply moisturizing cream to wet face and massage face thoroughly.
7. Apply eye cream.
8. Blot off excess cream.
9. Spray face lightly with mineral water and let dry naturally.

Weekly Routine

1. Cleanse face as usual with cleansing cream.
2. Optional wash with soap and water.
3. Follow with skin freshener.
4. Apply moisturizing cream and eye cream.
5. Steam face for five to ten minutes.
6. Remove cream with skin freshener.
7. Apply beauty mask of your choice and leave on for amount of time specified in recipe.
8. Remove mask and rinse face thoroughly. Pat dry.
9. Apply skin freshener.
10. Apply moisturizing cream. Massage deeply, but gently.
11. Apply eye cream.

12. Blot off excess cream.

13. Spray face lightly with mineral water and let dry naturally.

Monthly Facial

1. Cleanse face as usual with cleansing cream.

2. Optional wash with soap and water.

3. Follow with skin freshener.

4. Apply eye cream.

5. Apply moisturizing cream to entire face and throat (including eye area, over eye cream). Massage thoroughly.

6. Steam face for five to ten minutes.

7. Remove creams with skin freshener.

8. Apply warm vegetable oil of your choice to entire face and throat.

9. Cover face with warm, wet washcloth and lie down to rest for ten minutes.

10. Remove oil with skin freshener.

11. Apply a defoliating or superficial peeling beauty mask. Place cotton pads soaked in rosewater or witch hazel over eyes.

12. Lie down and rest for specified time.

13. Remove mask and rinse face thoroughly. Pat dry.

14. Pat skin freshener smartly onto face with fingertips. Slap-pat repeatedly until face is dry.

15. Apply moisturizing cream. Massage deeply.

16. Apply eye cream.

17. Blot off excess cream.

18. Spray face lightly with mineral or rose water and let dry naturally.

ANTI-AGE ROUTINES FOR OILY SKIN

Morning Routine

1. Lay two applications of warm, wet washcloth over face to open pores.

2. Smooth cleansing cream over face. Remove with washcloth (clean washcloth daily).

3. With mild soap, wash face thoroughly. Rinse well and pat dry.

4. With short, firm strokes upward and outward, cleanse entire face with cotton pads moistened with skin freshener. Use fresh cotton as needed and cleanse until pad it free of dirt.

5. Apply protection cream lightly. Do not massage.

6. Apply eye cream.

7. Completely blot off excess cream.

Midday Touchup

1. Keep "crinkle stick" (recipe in chapter 3) or small pot of petroleum jelly in your bag, and when you repair your makeup during the day, pat stick gently over any wrinkled area (right over makeup) around the eyes, mouth, etc.

2. With dry tissue or cotton ball and skin freshener, blot excess oil and/or grime from face.

Evening Routine

1. Apply cleansing cream over entire face. Gently but firmly remove makeup with several clean tissues.

2. Apply cleansing cream for a second time and remove with washcloth.

3. Wash face with soap as prescribed in morning routine.

4. Remove any remaining dirt or makeup with skin freshener.

5. Apply eye cream.

6. Apply protection cream.

7. Blot off excess cream completely.

Once- or Twice-Weekly Routine

1. Cleanse face as usual with cleansing cream.

2. Wash face as usual with soap.

3. Follow with skin freshener.

4. Steam face *gently* for ten minutes.

5. Apply beauty mask of your choice and leave on for amount of time specified in recipe or purchased product.

6. Remove mask and rinse face thoroughly. Pat dry.

7. Apply skin freshener.

8. Apply eye cream.

9. Apply protection cream.

10. Blot off any excess cream completely.

Monthly Facial

1. Cleanse face as usual with cleansing cream.

2. Wash face as usual with soap.

3. Follow with skin freshener.

4. Apply protection cream to face. Cover face with wet, warm washcloth and lie down to rest for five minutes.

5. Remove cream with skin freshener.

6. Steam face for ten minutes. Pat dry.

7. Apply a defoliating or superficial peeling beauty mask. Place cotton pads soaked in rose water or witch hazel over eyes.

8. Lie down and rest for specified time.

9. Remove mask and rinse face thoroughly. Pat dry.

10. Apply skin freshener.

11. Apply protection cream.*

12. Apply eye cream.

13. Blot off any excess cream completely.

ANTI-AGE ROUTINES FOR COMBINATION SKIN

Morning Routine

1. Lay several applications of warm, wet washcloth over face to open pores.

2. Smooth a mineral-oil-based cleansing cream over face. Massage well only on normal or dry areas. Remove with washcloth (clean washcolth daily).

3. This step is optional, but if you want to wash with soap and water, now is the time.

4. With short, firm strokes upward and outward, cleanse face with cotton pads moistened with the appropriate skin fresheners (you'll need two lotions). Use fresh cotton as needed and cleanse until pad is free of dirt.

5. Apply a natural vegetable-oil-base moisturizing cream to entire face and massage normal or dry areas deeply.†

6. Apply eye cream.

7. Blot off excess cream from normal or dry areas and firmly wipe off cream from oily areas with a tissue (enough cream will remain to protect the oily areas under makeup or against the weather without adding extra oils).

8. Spray dry areas of the face lightly with mineral water and let dry naturally.

Midday Touchup

1. Keep "crinkle stick" (recipe in chapter 3) or small pot of petroleum jelly in your bag, and when you repair your makeup during the day, pat the stick gently over any wrinkled area (right over makeup) around the eyes, mouth, etc.

* See note on page 53.
† See note on page 53.

2. Blot off any excess oil or grime with dry tissue. (You can blot oily areas lightly with a pad moistened with skin freshener.)

Evening Routine

1. Apply cleansing cream over entire face. Gently but firmly remove makeup with several clean tissues.

2. Lay several applications of warm, wet washcloth over entire face to open pores.

3. Apply cleansing cream for a second time and remove with washcloth.

4. Optional wash with soap and water.

5. Remove any remaining dirt or makeup with skin fresheners.

6. Apply moisturizing cream to entire face and massage normal or dry areas thoroughly.†

7. Apply eye cream.

8. Blot off excess cream from normal or dry areas and wipe cream off oily areas with a tissue.

9. Spray dry areas of face lightly with mineral water and let dry naturally.

Weekly Routine

1. Cleanse face as usual with cleansing cream.

2. Optional wash with soap and water.

3. Follow with skin fresheners.

4. Steam face for ten minutes (recipes in chapter 3).

5. Prepare only half recipe for a mask for oily skin and half recipe for a mask for normal or dry skin. Apply beauty masks to appropriate sections of face and leave on for amount of time specified in recipes.

6. Remove masks and rinse face thoroughly. Pat dry.

7. Apply skin freshener to oily areas.

8. Apply moisturizing cream to entire face and massage normal or dry areas deeply.†

9. Apply eye cream.

10. Blot off excess cream from normal or dry areas and wipe cream off oily areas with a tissue.

11. Spray dry areas of face lightly with mineral water and let dry normally.

† See note on page 53.

Monthly Facial

1. Cleanse face as usual with cleansing cream.
2. Optional wash with soap and water.
3. Follow with skin fresheners.
4. Apply moisturizing cream to normal or dry areas only. Massage thoroughly.
5. Cover face with warm, wet washcloth and lie down to rest for ten minutes *or* steam face for ten minutes.
6. Remove cream with skin freshener.
7. Apply an appropriate defoliating or superficial peeling beauty mask to each skin-type area. Place cotton pads soaked in rosewater or witch hazel over eyes.
8. Lie down and rest for specified time.
9. Remove masks and rinse face thoroughly. Pat dry.
10. Apply skin fresheners to oily areas.
11. Apply moisturizing cream to entire face and massage normal or dry areas deeply.†
12. Apply eye cream.
13. Blot off excess cream from normal or dry areas and wipe cream off oily areas with a tissue.
14. Spray dry areas of face lightly with mineral water and let dry naturally.

ANTI-AGE ROUTINES FOR AGING SKIN

Morning Routine

1. Wet face with warm water and smooth cleansing cream over face. Massage gently. Place warm, wet washcloth (clean washcloth daily) over face two or three times. Remove cream with washcloth, fingers or complexion brush, using washing motion if cream contains beauty grains.
2. With short, firm strokes upward and outward, cleanse entire face with cotton balls moistened in skin freshener. Use fresh cotton as needed and cleanse until pad is free of dirt.
3. Again place warm, wet washcloth over face two or three times and leave face wet. Apply moisturizing cream and massage gently onto wet face. Place warm, wet washcloth over face one last time.
4. Apply eye cream.
5. Blot off any excess cream.
6. Spray face lightly with mineral or rosewater and let dry naturally.

† See note on page 53.

Midday Touchup

1. Keep "crinkle stick" (recipe in chapter 3) or small pot of petroleum jelly in your bag, and when you repair your makeup during the day, pat the stick gently over any wrinkled area (right over makeup) around eyes, mouth, etc. Be sure to smooth out any makeup that may have found its way into crevices.

2. Blot off any grime with a tissue lightly moistened with warm water.

Evening Routine

1. Apply vegetable oil over entire face. Gently but firmly remove makeup with several clean tissues.

2. Apply cleansing cream and remove as in morning routine.

3. Remove any remaining dirt or makeup with skin freshener.

4. Place warm, wet washcloth over face two or three times. Spray face lightly with mineral water. Apply moisturizing cream and massage gently but thoroughly. Place warm, wet washcloth over face one more time.

5. Apply eye cream.

6. Blot off any excess cream.

7. Spray face lightly with mineral or rosewater and let dry naturally.

Weekly Routine

1. Cleanse face as usual with vegetable oil or cleansing cream.

2. Follow with skin freshener.

3. Wet face with warm water and apply moisturizing cream and eye cream on wet face.

4. Steam face for five minutes (recipe in chapter 3).

5. Remove creams with skin freshener.

6. Apply beauty mask of your choice and leave on for amount of time specified in recipe.

7. Remove mask and rinse face thoroughly. Pat dry.

8. Place warm, wet washcloth over face two or three times. Spray face lightly with mineral water. Apply moisturizing cream and massage thoroughly.

9. Apply eye cream.

10. Blot off any excess cream.

11. Spray face lightly with mineral or rosewater and let dry naturally.

Monthly Facial

1. Cleanse face as usual with vegetable oil or cleansing cream.

2. Optional soap and water wash.

3. Follow with skin freshener.

4. Apply eye cream.

5. Wet face with warm water. Apply moisturizing cream to entire (wet) face and throat (including eye area over eye cream). Massage thoroughly.

6. Steam face for five minutes.

7. Remove creams with skin freshener.

8. Wet face with warm water. Apply warm vegetable oil of your choice to entire wet face and throat.

9. Cover face with warm, wet washcloth and lie down to rest for ten minutes.

10. Remove oil with skin freshener.

11. Apply a defoliating beauty mask. Place cotton pads soaked in rosewater or witch hazel over eyes.

12. Lie down and rest for specified time for mask.

13. Remove mask and rinse face thoroughly. Pat dry.

14. Wet face with warm water. Apply moisturizing cream over wet face and massage thoroughly.

15. Apply eye cream.

16. Blot off any excess cream.

17. Spray face with mineral or rosewater and let dry naturally.

Notes

If your skin is excessively oily, use the protection cream only when you are intending to apply makeup or to subject your skin to the dirt and grime of outdoor air. If you are going to remain in the house or go to bed, try leaving the skin free of any cream except eye cream. Your natural oils may be enough to keep the skin lubricated. If not, apply a protection cream every time you cleanse your skin.

† If the oily areas are excessively oily, use moisturizing cream on those areas only when you are intending to apply makeup or to subject your skin to the dirt and grime of outdoor weather. If you are going to remain in the house or go to bed, try leaving the oily areas free of any cream. Always be sure to apply moisturizing cream to normal or dry areas. (Another alternative is to make up a batch of protection cream for oily skin and use that on the oily areas.)

Tips on Your Monthly Facial for All Types of Skin

The monthly routines described previously for each individual skin type are complete home facials. A few general tips, however, can provide further explanation and add to the procedure. As a part of all facials for all skin types, you will notice that after cleansing, you begin your facial with a relaxing and beneficial steambath for your face. The reason for this is that the warmth of the steam opens the pores, unclogs them and encourages toxins to be eliminated externally—all of which is necessary for the hygiene of your skin.

I do not recommend dry heat, however (such as a sauna). It does cause the skin to perspire and eliminate impurities, but it can also cause the skin to become dehydrated. Water is one of the most precious commodities the skin requires; steam heat offers the gentle warmth necessary to purge the system of poisons and at the same time surrounds the skin with hydrating water particles.

That's gentle heat. Never subject your skin to hot *anything*. It will only weaken the elasticity of your skin.

A five- or ten-minute steam, depending on your skin type, with one of the steam soups from the recipe section in chapter 3 should serve you well. There are a couple of ways to go about it.

If you have a vaporizer (there are some manufactured especially for this purpose), simply add your steam soup in the prescribed amount and steam away, unless your vaporizer specifically recommends only the use of plain water. Or you can heat the soup in a pot, *remove it from heat* and cover your head, and the entire opening of the vessel, with a towel to keep the steam in. It's easy either way.

Next, pat your face dry with a soft towel and apply the mask you have prepared in advance. And now let me prepare *you* in advance. Beauty masks can be messy. I suggest you wear nothing at all from the waist up; however, if you must wear something, make it a plastic cape or an old towel pinned around your shoulder.

Pin your hair up and keep the little wisps away from your face with a turban or a headband.

A man's shaving brush is a nice, professional method of applying soupier masks, but your fingers work just as well.

If your skin is extremely thin or sensitive, stay away from abrasive masks, like those containing oatmeal or almonds, and the strong pulling masks, such as egg white or mint. Do not apply masks over an open wound and, in all cases, do not cover the eye area with a mask. Pat some honey (a good natural moisturizer) under your eyes while the mask is on your face.

If you have any blackheads or whiteheads, you may clean your pores after removing the mask. *Caution must be taken when emptying clogged pores.* Take a tissue and tear it in half. Cover both index fingers and press gently but firmly on either side of the blemish. Only remove that substance that dislodges without effort. *Do not apply great pressure.* Re-cover the fingers with a clean section of the tissue for each separate removal. (Do not squeeze any sort of blemish on the nose. If this is done improperly, you can break capillaries, which will result in a rather permanent redness. If infection ensues, it can drain directly to the brain and prove fatal. If you have persistent bumps on the nose, see a dermatologist.)

When the face is clean, wipe it gently with a cotton pad moistened with witch hazel or your regular skin freshener to disinfect the area. If you have an actual eruption (as opposed to tiny imperfections hiding just under the skin, which are easily removed) do not apply cream or makeup of any sort to it. If you wish, cover it with a drying agent to aid the healing process.

Any minor impurities will be coaxed to the surface by the drawing power of a mask. If you're persistent in regular home facials, I think you'll find that even obvious blemish problems will eventually diminish, if not disappear altogether.

Your Body Skin—How to Give Yourself a "Body" Facial

We have seen already that as we get older, face skin begins to require special care to help it slough off its dead skin cell layer in order to gain a youthful appearance. The same is true of the skin covering our entire body. When body skin is young, the simple brisk rubbing with a towel after bathing is enough to keep the skin smooth and polished. But with age, a bit more effort is in order.

Body facials are fast and easy, but they are very messy, so I suggest that you stand in a tub or shower after you bathe; that way, you can just rinse the defoliating materials down the drain after you are finished. Since the recipes for these superficial peelers are the same for all types of body skins, I will give them here.

Sesame and the Sea Body Peeler

In a bowl, mix 1 pint sesame oil with ½ cup sea salt. (You can buy pulverized salt, or, if you get the whole kernels, pulverize them in your blender.) Stand under a warm shower (your body should be freshly washed) for five minutes in order to soften the skin; cut off the shower and scoop handfuls of the oil and salt into your hand and rub gently but firmly with repeated strokes over your entire body. Sea salt is very abrasive, so be careful; you want only to remove the top layer of dead skin cells. Spend extra effort on elbows, heels, knees and feet. Use a back brush covered with the mixture on your back. You will see a marvelous rosy hue come to your body as it achieves a young, polished shine. Your body skin is benefiting from the same internal cleansing as your facial skin during a face facial. When you are finished, rinse well with warm water, pat dry with a big, thirsty towel and moisturize your entire body skin with sesame oil. You will feel pampered beyond belief.

Almond-Oatmeal Superficial Body Peeler

Mix ½ cup pulverized almonds (pulverized in your blender), ½ cup pulverized steel-ground oatmeal and 1 cup olive oil in a bowl. This is a gentler body facial than the sea salt recipe above and is recommended especially for older skins. Follow application instructions as outlined in previous recipe.

Oatmeal Body Scrub

Pulverize steel-ground oatmeal in your blender. One cup should be enough. Stand in the tub or shower after cleansing your body and dry yourself thoroughly. Now rub the oatmeal vigorously over every inch of your body skin, paying special attention to elbows, heels, knees and feet (you can do your face at the same time if you wish), until you see a rosy hue and feel a polished finish to your skin. Rinse in warm water. Towel-dry gently and moisturize entire body with sesame oil. Rub oil in completely; a little goes a long way.

Your Body Skin on a Daily Basis

The skin of your body needs moisturizing for the same reasons your facial skin needs moisturizing. It does not require as much care, however, because it is not customarily exposed to the elements (and makeup) as is your face. Each day, after your bath or shower, massage your body well with a small amount of sesame oil. Massage deeply to bring the blood to the surface on all areas except your breasts. Since sesame is a natural vegetable oil, it will penetrate after a few moments, thus avoiding any stain on your clothes, and it will keep your skin soft and protected all day. Adding some of your favorite perfume oil to the sesame is a very effective method of retaining the fragrance throughout the day.

3

PRIVATE-LABEL COSMETICS

Now that you understand what the skin is all about and what is required by its nature for its health and beauty, you may wish, as I do, to make your own skin-care products. The biggest reason for doing this—aside from the large amount of money to be saved—is that only by creating your own custom cosmetics can you know exactly how much of what you are putting on your skin . . . and why. You know that the ingredients used in your own private labels are there for a reason (you even know what the reasons are), and you know that they are fresh and pure and natural. You also gain complete allergy control by making your own products since, knowing precisely the ingredients and their amounts, you can isolate any allergic reaction (in the unlikely event you should suffer one) in a knowledgeable and methodical manner by simply eliminating the ingredient causing the reaction from all future products.

It has been my experience that once a woman begins to make her own skin-care treatments, she seldom again considers buying them. Once you have control of this issue, you begin to feel very vulnerable leaving the subject up to anyone else's judgment.

The Making of Creams

As we discussed in chapter 2, the oils used in your creams are determined by your individual skin type. Therefore, the recipes that follow will specify mineral oils for oily skins and vegetable and animal oils (lanolin only) for dry skins. Normal skins are included under the dry skin categories, but if you fall into this category, you can really select any recipes you wish, depending upon whether or not you feel the need of a penetrating cream.

The other ingredients are essentially the same. Honey beeswax can be ordered from your druggist if he doesn't already carry it or purchased at farmers' markets and country fairs (look for the person selling honey). Natural beeswax is preferable to paraffin (found in the grocery store), which is used in most commercial products, because it will not clog pores. However, if you absolutely cannot find beeswax, you can substitute paraffin as a second choice and be no worse off than if you purchased a cream ready-made. The water portion of each recipe will call for witch hazel (except in the case of aging skins), which is always available and pure; however, you may substitute rosewater or any flavor of extract or freshly strained fruit juices to provide variety and lovely scents to your creams if you wish. The borax called for in each recipe simply acts as an emulsifier to hold the other ingredients together. It, on its own merit, is also a skin softener. Lecithin is called for in dry skin moisturizing creams because it acts to help the natural oils penetrate the skin.

The making of creams is really very simple. You know now that they are basically a combination of waxes, oils and water. As a general rule for preparation, just remember that the waxes are melted together first (over *low* heat), the oils warmed and beaten into the waxes and the heated water dribbled slowly and beaten into that mixture. And that's all there is to it. Once you've gathered the ingredients together, it will take approximately five to ten minutes from start to finish.

Homemade creams will vary in consistency. It's really a matter of personal preference whether you want a soft or firm cream; the important factor is what's *in* the cream. Sometimes the consistency will firm slightly after the cream sits for a few hours. If this happens, simply rewhip the cream lightly with a fork and it will then remain soft and fluffy.

After you make one of these creams for the first time, if you'd like to change its texture, you can. Simply add more beeswax if you want it firmer, more water if you want it thinner. If you wish to change the scent, use any flavor extract as mentioned earlier. (When heating extracts, use a *low* heat.)

If waxes harden on spoons or in pots, heat the utensil over boiling water and, when the wax is melted again, wash quickly with hot, soapy water and a steel-wool pad. The way to avoid this is to wash pots and spoons by the same method immediately after using them and pre-measure your wax.

Because beeswax usually comes in cake form, it's more convenient to melt it down and measure it out in advance than to melt and measure for each individual recipe. Cut some aluminum foil into four-to six-inch squares. Form a little cup out of each square and set the little cups in a row on the counter top. Next, melt a cake or two of beeswax (over *low* heat) and measure 1 teaspoon of the liquid wax into each cup. When the wax hardens, wrap the rest of the cup around the wax and simply store your little balls of wax in a box until you need them. If a recipe calls for 2 teaspoons of wax, unwrap two balls and melt them down again. If it calls for 1 tablespoon, unwrap three balls, and so on.

Another method for measuring solid waxes or fats—such as cocoa butter or coconut oil—is to use water, a measuring cup and the principle of displacement. Example: If the recipe calls for 1 ounce of cocoa butter, fill a measuring cup with 1 ounce of water. Drop some cocoa butter into the water and keep adding more of it, a little at a time, until the water level reaches 2 ounces. Then pour out the water. The remaining cocoa butter will measure 1 ounce when melted down.

You'll notice that whenever perishable ingredients are included in the recipe, I specify refrigeration. It is true that if you cool these creams, they will last longer. I, however, do not refrigerate mine and most of them last for months, certainly long enough to use them up. Be sure your hands are clean before dipping fingers into anything made without preservatives that goes on your face to avoid adding unwanted bacteria.

If you wish to include vitamins in your homemade creams, simply puncture a few vitamin A, D or E capsules and empty the contents into your cream at the end of the beating procedure, when the cream is completely formed and cool. I do not think there is much value in this addition, but if you are convinced that you want vitamin creams, you will at least save a good deal of money by making your own.

Vitamins are necessary for your skin, surely, but from the *inside* via the blood, as you learned in chapter 2. This is the only method of nourishing or feeding the skin. An internal vitamin deficiency will be reflected in the surface quality of the skin. However, although experiments have shown that these particular vitamins can be absorbed in minute amounts by topical application to the surface of the skin, common sense alone will tell you that the process has little, if any, value. Think of the small amount of vitamin substances included (either by you or by a commercial company) in a jar of cream. Then think of the tiny bit of cream you put on your finger and then think of *that* small amount being spread out over your entire face. Even if the idea had value, which I don't think it does, it could hardly do much good in such small amounts.

I have, however, included a vitamin-E cream for each skin type, that vitamin being present in the wheat germ oil included in this particular recipe. There is no real, irrefutable scientific evidence that this vitamin offers any more benefits than any other oil, but I personally know some people who through their own direct—nonscientific—experimentation have had positive results through inclusion of this vitamin in their skin-care regimes. Others, myself among them, experience adverse reactions. But for those of you with skin that might be able to benefit from the application of vitamin E, the cream is here for you to try without the greater financial investment involved in *buying* a promise.

As for the beating of creams, an electric hand mixer is easiest, but any other method of hand beating works just as well.

One last word on cleansing and moisturizing or protection creams. If you wish neither to purchase expensive creams nor make your own, you can with complete confidence use only the pure oils, by themselves, for these purposes. If you have oily skin, simply apply either mineral oil or petroleum jelly in each case. If you have dry skin, use any vegetable oil of your choice or combine several together in one pretty bottle. (Sesame or almond oil are particularly nice if you choose to use only one oil "straight.") Dry skins can also use plain vegetable shortening or margarine as cleansing cream, since they are hydrogenated oils already hardened into a cream consistency for you.

Now, on to some recipes.

RECIPES FOR CLEANSING CREAMS
FOR NORMAL AND DRY SKINS

(Remember, whatever vegetable oil is called for in these recipes, you can substitute any other natural vegetable oil of your choice.)

Cocoa Butter Cleansing Cream

1 *tablespoon beeswax*
1 *ounce cocoa butter*
1 *ounce safflower oil*
1 *ounce almond oil*
2 *ounces witch hazel*
¼ *teaspoon borax*

Melt beeswax over *low* heat. Melt cocoa butter separately and add to other warmed oils. Dribble oils into beeswax, beating constantly. Warm witch hazel and borax and beat into first mixture. Beat until creamy and cool. Makes 3 ounces. Refrigerate.

Coconut Cleansing Cream

2 *teaspoons beeswax*
2 *ounces coconut oil*
2 *ounces almond oil*
2 *ounces witch hazel*
     (or coconut-flavored extract)
¼ *teaspoon borax*

Melt beeswax over low heat. Heat and combine coconut oil and almond oil and beat into wax. Dissolve borax in hot witch hazel and, dribbling slowly, beat into wax and oil mixture until cool, creamy consistency is achieved. Makes 5 ounces. Refrigerate.

Ultra-Rich Cleansing Cream

2 *teaspoons beeswax*
3 *ounces anhydrous lanolin*
2 *ounces olive oil*
3 *ounces witch hazel*
¼ *teaspoon borax*

Melt beeswax over low heat. Melt and heat together lanolin and olive oil and beat well into wax. Heat witch hazel and borax and dribble slowly into mixture, beating all the while, until it is cool and creamy. Makes 5 ounces. Refrigerate.

Almond Defoliating Cleansing Cream

3 *tablespoons almonds*
2 *teaspoons beeswax*
3 *ounces almond oil*
¼ *teaspoon borax*
2 *ounces witch hazel*
      (*or almond-flavored extract*)

Pulverize almonds in blender and set aside. Melt beeswax over low heat. Heat almond oil and beat into wax. Dissolve borax in witch hazel and, pouring slowly, beat well into mixture until cool, creamy consistency is reached. Stir in pulverized almonds until well blended. After applying this cream, use fingers with circular motions, as if washing the face, in order to remove dead skin cells via the abrasiveness of the almonds before tissuing or washing off. Makes 4 ounces. Refrigerate.

RECIPES FOR MOISTURIZING CREAMS FOR NORMAL AND DRY SKINS

Vitamin-E Moisturizing Cream

1 *tablespoon beeswax*
3 *ounces wheat germ oil*
      (*do not substitute any other oil*)
1 *ounce cocoa butter*
1 *ounce liquid lecithin*
3 *ounces witch hazel*
¼ *teaspoon borax*

Melt beeswax over low heat. Combine and heat wheat germ oil with cocoa butter. After this is heated, stir in lecithin and beat oil mixture into wax. Heat witch hazel and borax and pour slowly into mixture, beating all the while, until cool and creamy. Makes 5 ounces. Refrigerate.

Deep-Penetrating Moisturizing Cream

2 *teaspoons beeswax*
3 *tablespoons anhydrous lanolin*
1 *ounce sesame oil*

1 ounce lecithin
3 ounces witch hazel
¼ teaspoon borax

Melt beeswax over low heat. Melt lanolin and sesame oil together and then stir in lecithin before beating oil mixture into melted wax. Heat witch hazel and borax and beat, dribbling slowly, into first mixture until cool and creamy. Makes 5 ounces. Refrigerate.

Blend of Oils Moisturizing Cream

1 tablespoon beeswax
1 ounce avocado oil
1 ounce sesame oil
1 ounce soy oil
1 ounce olive oil
1 ounce liquid lecithin
¼ teaspoon borax
2 ounces witch hazel

Melt beeswax over low heat. Combine and heat all oils, stir in lecithin and beat mixture into beeswax. Combine and heat borax with witch hazel and, dribbling slowly, beat into mixture until cool and creamy. Makes 5 ounces. Refrigerate.

Sesame-Almond Moisturizing Cream

1 tablespoon beeswax
2 ounces sesame oil
2 ounces almond oil
1 tablespoon anhydrous lanolin
1 tablespoon liquid lecithin
¼ teaspoon borax
4 ounces witch hazel

Melt beeswax over low heat. Melt and combine oils with lanolin and then stir in lecithin. Beat oil mixture into melted wax. Heat borax and witch hazel and, pouring slowly, beat into mixture until cool and creamy. Makes 6 ounces. Refrigerate.

RECIPES FOR CLEANSING CREAMS FOR OILY SKIN

Coconut Cleansing Cream

2 teaspoons beeswax
2 ounces coconut oil (melted)
1 ounce mineral oil
2 ounces witch hazel
     (or coconut-flavored extract)
¼ ounce borax

Melt beeswax over low heat. Heat and combine coconut oil and mineral oil and beat into wax. Dissolve borax in heated witch hazel and, dribbling slowly, beat into mixture until cool and creamy consistency is achieved. Makes 4 ounces.

Ultra-Rich Cleansing Cream

1 tablespoon beeswax
3 ounces petroleum jelly
2 ounces mineral oil
3 ounces witch hazel
¼ teaspoon borax

Melt beeswax over low heat. Melt and heat together petroleum jelly and mineral oil and beat well into wax. Heat witch hazel and borax and dribble slowly, while beating continuously, into mixture until cool and creamy. Makes 5 ounces.

Cocoa Butter Cleansing Cream

1 tablespoon beeswax
1 ounce cocoa butter
1 ounce petroleum jelly
1 ounce mineral oil
2 ounces witch hazel
¼ teaspoon borax

Melt beeswax over low heat. Melt cocoa butter separately and add to warmed and melted petroleum jelly and mineral oil. Heat oil mixtures into wax. Warm witch hazel with borax and, dribbling slowly, beat into mixture until cool and creamy. Makes 4 ounces.

Defoliating Oatmeal Cleansing Cream

3 *tablespoons steel-ground oatmeal*
2 *teaspoons beeswax*
3 *ounces mineral oil*
¼ *teaspoon borax*
2 *ounces witch hazel*

Pulverize oatmeal in blender and set aside. Melt beeswax over low heat. Heat mineral oil and beat into wax. Dissolve borax in heated witch hazel and, pouring slowly, beat into mixture until cool and creamy. Stir in pulverized oatmeal until well blended. After applying this cream, use fingers, washing the face with circular motions in order to utilize the abrasive aspects of the oatmeal to rid the skin of dead cells, then tissue off or wash off as usual. Makes 4 ounces.

RECIPES FOR PROTECTION CREAMS FOR OILY SKIN

Vitamin-E Protection Cream

1 *tablespoon beeswax*
1 *ounce petroleum jelly*
1 *ounce wheat germ oil*
    (do not substitute any other oil)
2 *ounces mineral oil*
3 *ounces witch hazel*
¼ *teaspoon borax*

Melt beeswax over low heat. Melt petroleum jelly with two other oils and beat into wax. Heat witch hazel and borax and, dribbling slowly, beat into mixture until cool and creamy. Makes 5 ounces.

Extra-Protection Protection Cream

2 *teaspoons beeswax*
3 *ounces petroleum jelly*
2 *ounces witch hazel*
¼ *teaspoon borax*

Melt beeswax over low heat. Melt petroleum jelly and beat into wax. Heat witch hazel and borax and, pouring slowly, beat into mixture until cool and creamy. Makes 3 ounces.

Light-Coverage Protection Cream

1 *tablespoon beeswax*
2 *ounces mineral oil*
1 *ounce witch hazel (or 1 tablespoon witch*
  hazel and 1 tablespoon strained cucumber
  juice is especially nice)
¼ *teaspoon borax*

Melt beeswax over low heat. Heat mineral oil and beat into wax. Heat witch hazel (or mixture with cucumber juice) with borax and, dribbling slowly, beat into mixture until cool and creamy. Makes 3 ounces.

Protein Protection Cream

1 *tablespoon beeswax*
1 *ounce coconut oil*
1 *ounce mineral oil*
1 *ounce petroleum jelly*
1 *teaspoon alcohol*
1 *ounce witch hazel*
¼ *teaspoon borax*
1 *egg yolk*

Melt beeswax over low heat. Melt and beat together the coconut oil, mineral oil and petroleum jelly and beat into wax. Heat alcohol, witch hazel and borax and, dribbling slowly, beat into mixture until cool and creamy. Beat egg yolk until lemon yellow in color and beat into cream. Makes approximately 4 ounces. *Definitely refrigerate.*

RECIPES FOR CLEANSING CREAMS FOR AGING SKINS
(Do not substitute oils)

(Rosewater is recommended rather than the usual witch hazel for creams designed for an aging skin, as it is gentler.)

Cocoa Butter Cleansing Cream

2 *teaspoons beeswax*
2 *ounces cocoa butter*
1 *ounce olive oil*
2 *ounces rosewater*
¼ *teaspoon borax*

Melt beeswax over low heat. Melt cocoa butter and heat with olive oil. Beat oil mixture into wax. Heat rosewater with borax and, dribbling slowly, beat into mixture until cool and creamy. Makes 3 ounces. Refrigerate.

Coconut Cleansing Cream

2 *teaspoons beeswax*
2 *ounces coconut oil (melted)*
1 *ounce sesame oil*
2 *tablespoons anhydrous lanolin*
2 *ounces rosewater*
¼ *teaspoon borax*

Melt beeswax over low heat. Melt, combine and heat coconut oil, sesame oil and lanolin and beat this oil mixture into the wax. Heat rosewater with borax and, pouring slowly, beat into mixture until cool and creamy. Makes 4 ounces. Refrigerate.

Almond Defoliating Cleansing Cream

3 *tablespoons almonds*
1 *tablespoon beeswax*
2 *ounces almond oil*
2 *tablespoons anhydrous lanolin*
¼ *teaspoon borax*
3 *ounces rosewater*

Pulverize almonds in blender and set aside. Melt beeswax over low heat. Heat almond oil and lanolin and beat into wax. Dissolve borax in rosewater and, dribbling slowly, beat into mixture until cool and creamy. Stir in pulverized almonds until cream is well blended. After applying cream, use fingers in a circular motion to *gently* wash the face in order to rid the surface of dead skin cells and then remove cream as usual. Makes 4 ounces. Refrigerate.

Oatmeal Defoliating Cleansing Cream

3 *tablespoons steel-ground oatmeal*
1 *tablespoon beeswax*
1 *ounce cocoa butter*
2 *ounces olive oil*
¼ *teaspoon borax*
1 *ounce rosewater*

Pulverize oatmeal in blender and set aside. Melt beeswax over low heat. Melt and combine heated cocoa butter and olive oil and beat into wax. Dissolve borax in heated rosewater and, pouring slowly, beat into mixture until cool and creamy. Beat in oatmeal until cream is well blended. After applying cream, use fingers in a circular motion to *gently* wash the face in order to rid the surface of dead skin cells and then remove cream as usual. Makes 3 ounces. Refrigerate.

RECIPES FOR MOISTURIZING CREAMS FOR AGING SKIN
(Do not substitute oils)

Vitamin-E Moisturizing Cream

1 *tablespoon beeswax*
2 *tablespoons anhydrous lanolin*
3 *ounces wheat germ oil*
1 *ounce liquid lecithin*
¼ *teaspoon borax*
3 *ounces rosewater*

Melt beeswax over low heat. Melt and heat lanolin with wheat germ oil, stir in lecithin and beat mixture into wax. Dissolve borax in rosewater and, dribbling slowly, beat into mixture until cool and creamy. Makes 5 ounces. Refrigerate.

Deep-Penetrating Moisturizing Cream

2 *teaspoons beeswax*
4 *tablespoons anhydrous lanolin*
1 *ounce olive oil*
1 *ounce liquid lecithin*
¼ *teaspoon borax*
3 *ounces rosewater*

Melt beeswax over low heat. Melt lanolin and heat with olive oil, stir in lecithin and beat mixture into wax. Dissolve borax in heated rosewater and, pouring slowly, beat into mixture until cool and creamy. Makes 6 ounces. Refrigerate.

Ultra-Rich Moisturizing Cream

1 ounce cocoa butter
1 ounce castor oil
3 tablespoons anhydrous lanolin
1 ounce wheat germ oil
1 ounce liquid lecithin
1 ounce olive oil

Heat all together (do not be concerned if mixture becomes foamy), and beat until well blended. Makes approximately 6 ounces. Refrigerate.

Protein Moisturizing Cream

1 tablespoon beeswax
2 tablespoons anhydrous lanolin
1 ounce wheat germ oil
1 ounce almond or sesame oil
1 teaspoon liquid lecithin
¼ teaspoon borax
1 ounce rosewater
1 egg yolk

Melt beeswax over low heat. Melt and heat together lanolin and oils, stir in lecithin and beat mixture into wax. Dissolve borax into heated rosewater and, dribbling slowly, beat into mixture until cool and creamy. Beat egg yolk until lemon yellow in color and then beat into cream until well blended. Makes 3 ounces plus. *Definitely refrigerate.*

Skin Fresheners

These lotions have many different names: skin toners or tonics, conditioners, astringents, cleansing lotions, fresheners and texture lotions are a few of them. They are used after a cleansing cream for the specific purpose outlined in chapter 2. For oily skins, they are essential because they effectively remove any oils that may remain on the skin from a cleansing cream, even after a soap and water wash. And they are a vital part of any cleansing routine for all skin types because they tone and freshen the skin as well as stimulate circulation to promote, on a daily basis, that all-important internal cleansing examined in chapter 2. In addition, fresheners restore the skin's pH level to normal, should that be necessary, and tighten and close pores for a refined texture.

You'll hear those phrases repeated time and again: "tighten pores," "close enlarged pores." Actually, none of that really happens. True "pores," which are the minute openings of sweat glands, are hidden from the naked eye. They usually reach only the border between the dermis and the epidermis.

What is commonly thought of as a pore on the surface of the skin is actually an opening of the follicle of a baby hair, which you may or may not be able to see. Sometimes the openings grow naturally large in order to prepare not for a baby hair but for a large one. Then, if the large hair doesn't appear for some reason, you have an enlarged "pore."

Since the misnomer is solidly ingrained in beauty vocabulary, you will note that I, too, will misuse this term so as not to confuse you, and I shall refer to follicle openings as pores.

To be perfectly accurate, not only are the openings not pores that the lotions close and tighten, but the lotions don't actually "close" and "tighten" either. What actually happens is this: The slightly astringent qualities of the freshener cause the surrounding tissue to swell so that the tiny opening *seems* to be smaller—or "closed" and "tightened." This gives the skin that smooth, fine-grained texture so sought after by women of all skin types.

Application of skin fresheners is best done with cotton balls. Shake the bottle of lotion, hold the cotton over the opening until it is wet (not dripping), then, with firm movements to stimulate circulation, wipe the areas to be cleaned in an upward and outward motion. Use fresh cotton as needed. It's well to remember that you're not wiping the lotion *on*, you're wiping any leftover dirt *off*.

These fresheners are effective any time of the day for a quick cleanup or pick-me-up for the face. There are recipes for oily skins and dry skins as well as normal and aging skins. If you have a combination skin, simply make two appropriate lotions and use them accordingly.

For those of you who may be new to this type of lotion, I think you'll enjoy the fresh, clean feeling it imparts to your face. I believe that skin fresheners are the single most important cleaning agent you can use on your face.

RECIPES FOR SKIN FRESHENERS FOR NORMAL SKIN

Witch Hazel Lotion

1 *bottle witch hazel*

That's all. Just use this refreshing liquid by itself as you would any other fancier lotion.

Glycerin and Rosewater Lotion

4 ounces rosewater
½–1 ounce glycerin
1 ounce witch hazel

Shake together in bottle.

Fresh Fruit Skin Freshener

1 ounce any fresh fruit juice of your choice
 (strawberry, cucumber, lemon, grapefruit,
  etc.)
3 ounces witch hazel
1 ounce alcohol

Puree fresh fruit in blender (add a little witch hazel if needed) and strain well. Shake in pretty bottle with witch hazel and alcohol.

Chamomile Skin Freshener

3 ounces witch hazel
2 ounces chamomile tea
1 ounce alcohol

Shake together in pretty bottle.

Brandy Skin Freshener

4 ounces witch hazel
1 ounce brandy
1 ounce alcohol

Shake together in pretty bottle.

RECIPES FOR SKIN FRESHENERS FOR DRY SKIN

Strawberry or Cucumber Skin Freshener

1 *ounce either strawberry or cucumber juice*
    (do not use cucumber if skin is very dry)
4 *ounces witch hazel*
1 *teaspoon glycerin*

Puree strawberries or cucumbers in blender (add a little rosewater or witch hazel if some liquifying agent is necessary) and strain well. Shake in pretty bottle with witch hazel and glycerin.

Brandy Skin Freshener

4 *ounces witch hazel*
1 *ounce brandy*
1 *teaspoon glycerin*

Shake all together in pretty bottle.

Barley-Water Skin Freshener

¼ *cup barley*
1 *pint water*
4 *ounces witch hazel*
½ *ounce glycerin*

In saucepan, bring barley and water to boil. Lower heat and simmer for a half hour. Strain. When cool, add witch hazel and glycerin, bottle and keep in refrigerator. When using, apply as usual and follow with a cold-water rinse if you wish.

Chamomile Skin Freshener

4 *ounces witch hazel*
2 *ounces chamomile tea*
1 *teaspoon glycerin*

Shake together in pretty bottle.

RECIPES FOR SKIN FRESHENERS FOR OILY SKIN

Fresh Fruit Tonic Skin Freshener

2 ounces fresh fruit juice of your choice
   (lemon, grapefruit, strawberry, cucumber,
   etc.)
3 ounces witch hazel
2 ounces vodka

Puree fresh fruit in blender (add a little witch hazel if needed) and strain well. Shake together with other ingredients in pretty bottle.

Brandy Skin Freshener

3 ounces witch hazel
3 ounces brandy
1 ounce alcohol

Shake together in pretty bottle.

Witch Hazel Fizz Skin Freshener

4 ounces witch hazel
1 ounce alcohol
1 tablespoon camphor water
   (purchased in drugstore)
¼ teaspoon boric acid
1 teaspoon tincture of benzoin

Shake together in pretty bottle.

RECIPES FOR SKIN FRESHENERS FOR AGING SKIN

Strawberry or Cucumber Skin Freshener

1 ounce either strawberry or cucumber juice
   (do not use cucumber if skin is very dry)
4 ounces witch hazel
1 tablespoon vegetable oil

Puree strawberries or cucumbers in blender (use a little rosewater if needed to liquefy) and strain well. Shake together in pretty bottle with other ingredients.

Chamomile Skin Freshener

4 ounces witch hazel
3 ounces chamomile tea
1 tablespoon vegetable oil

Shake together in pretty bottle.

Rosewater Skin Freshener

3 ounces witch hazel
3 ounces rosewater
1 tablespoon vegetable oil

Shake together in pretty bottle.

Brandy Skin Freshener

4 ounces witch hazel
1 ounce brandy
1 tablespoon vegetable oil

Shake together in pretty bottle.

Eye Creams

The reasons the eye area wrinkles so easily are manifold. Firstly, the skin around the eye becomes naturally crinkled every time you laugh or smile or cry, so, after a certain number of years, lines appear simply from use. The skin in this area is also extremely thin and gets little, if any, circulation. And finally, there are no oil glands around the eye to keep the skin naturally lubricated.

An eye cream, because of the above realities, serves an entirely different function from that of any other type of cream you may use on your face. Since there are no sebaceous glands to stimulate, there is no need for a penetrating oil. In fact, eye creams should *not* penetrate, because the main reason for applying these creams is to keep the area moist and lubricated so that already existing lines will not deepen as quickly. Lines cannot be stopped, but they can be retarded to an amazing degree. Another purpose of an eye cream is to soften the skin and therefore diminish the *appearance* of lines. There are certain oils—castor oil, cocoa butter and coconut oil—that seem to aid in this effort. Do not misunderstand; creams made with these oils will not erase lines and wrinkles.

No beauty aid discovered or created so far has that magical power, and don't let anyone mislead you into thinking that any has. (Many of the new wrinkle and line "eraser" products temporarily tighten the area, but beware that they do not further dry out your skin as they tighten and, in the end, *increase* the actual lines.) What eye creams actually have the power to do is soften and moisturize.

During the day when you freshen your makeup, tap a "crinkle stick" (recipes follow) gently over the eye area to relubricate it. Plain petroleum jelly is one of the best eye creams available if you don't want to make a special one for yourself. Use it whenever you cleanse your face, and carry a small pot of it with you for touch-ups.

By the way, if you have an occasional bout of puffiness under your eyes when you get up in the morning due to lack of sleep, retention of water or overconsumption of alcohol, the following treatment will usually help the swelling disappear: Steep two tea bags in a cup of boiling water until the resulting tea is rather strong. Next, squeezing only enough liquid from the bags to keep them from dripping, put them in the freezer until they are very, very cold but not frozen. Squeeze them gently again to make sure the liquid tea is still wet on the surface, and then lie down, your feet higher than your head (put a couple of pillows under them), with one tea bag on each eye for ten to fifteen minutes. Puffiness will usually vanish completely with this method.

RECIPES FOR EYE CREAMS FOR ALL TYPES OF SKINS

Coconut Butter Eye Cream

1 teaspoon beeswax (optional)
1 tablespoon mineral oil
1 tablespoon petroleum jelly
1 tablespoon cocoa butter
1 tablespoon coconut oil
1 tablespoon castor oil

Melt beeswax over low heat (if included). Heat together all other ingredients and beat (into wax if used) together until cool. Makes about 2 ounces.

Vitamin-E Eye Cream

(Certain people have had luck with eye creams containing this vitamin; others—myself included—cannot use it at all as it makes

some eyes water. I include it here for those of you who wish to try it.)

> 2 *teaspoons beeswax*
> 1 *ounce mineral oil*
> 1 *ounce wheat germ oil*
> 1 *tablespoon petroleum jelly*

Melt beeswax over low heat. Heat other ingredients and beat into wax until cool and creamy. Makes 3 ounces.

Ultra-Rich Eye Cream

> 1 *tablespoon beeswax*
> 2 *tablespoons coconut oil*
> 1 *tablespoon castor oil*
> 2 *tablespoons petroleum jelly*
> 1 *ounce cocoa butter*
> 2 *tablespoons anhydrous lanolin*
>   *(used because it is sticky and keeps the*
>   *cream on the eye area, for those whose*
>   *eye creams seem to melt and run into*
>   *the eye itself)*
> 2 *ounces rosewater*
> ¼ *teaspoon borax*

Melt beeswax over low heat. Melt and heat oils, petroleum jelly, cocoa butter and lanolin together and beat into wax. Heat rosewater and borax and, pouring slowly, beat into mixture until cool and creamy. Makes 5 ounces.

CRINKLE STICKS

When you have finished preparing one of these crinkle stick creams, rotate the bottom of a well-cleaned, dry lipstick case until the inside portion reaches the top of the tube. Using your fingers, pack the cream into the case, pressing down firmly. When the cream is filled to the top, rotate the bottom of the tube downward to allow more room for packing. Continue this process until the tube is filled.

(Synthetic spermaceti, spermaceti being a wax from the head of a whale that is no longer legally possible to obtain, is used in these recipes in order to give the stick hardness and provide a slight stickiness that helps the product remain in place. It is available in your drugstore under the name Synerceti.)

Cocoa Butter Crinkle Stick

1 *ounce cocoa butter*
1 *teaspoon Synerceti*
1 *teaspoon heavy mineral oil*

Melt cocoa butter and Synerceti over low heat (in warm climates use 2 teaspoons Synerceti). Beat in warmed mineral oil and continue beating until cool. Scoop into small pot or lipstick case.

Slick Crinkle Stick

1 *tablespoon petroleum jelly*
1 *tablespoon cocoa butter*
1 *tablespoon castor oil*
1 *teaspoon beeswax*
½ *teaspoon Synerceti*

Melt all together over low heat and beat until cool. Scoop into small pot or lipstick case.

Beauty Masks

The various purposes for giving yourself a regular beauty mask and preceding its application with a steam tea were outlined in chapter 2; therefore, we can get right to recipes.

Chamomile Steam Tea for Normal, Dry and Aging Skins
(to open pores before application of a mask)

2 *quarts boiling water*
10 *chamomile tea bags*

Steep bags in water for one hour. Bring tea back to boil and remove from fire. Cover head with towel—creating a tent to keep in steam— and bend head (and clean face) over pot for ten minutes. (If you have an electronic steamer, you can make a much smaller amount of tea.) Save, as steam tea can be reused if kept in refrigerator.

Sage or Mint Steam Tea for Oily Skins
(to open pores before application of a mask)

Handful either dried mint or sage
2 *quarts boiling water*

Steep dried mint or sage in water for one hour. Strain. Bring tea back to boil and remove from fire. Cover head with a towel—creating a tent to keep in steam—and bend head (and clean face) over pot for ten minutes. (If you have an electronic steamer, you can make a much smaller amount of tea.) Save, as steam tea can be reused if kept in refrigerator.

RECIPES FOR BEAUTY MASKS FOR ANY TYPE SKIN

Bleaching Beauty Mask

2 *ounces buttermilk* or *plain yogurt*
2 *tablespoons whole wheat flour or wheat germ*

Blend milk or yogurt and flour into thick paste and apply to face. Leave on for twenty minutes and remove with warm water.

Protein Mask

1 *egg yolk*

Beat until lemon yellow in color and apply to clean face. Leave on for twenty minutes and remove with warm water. (Those with aging skins may want to mix in a little warm vegetable oil with egg yolk.)

Papaya Superficial Peeling or Defoliating Mask

¼ *fresh papaya*

Mash the fruit with a fork until smooth and apply to clean face. The natural enzymes in papaya consume, in a way, the dead layer of skin you are seeking to remove. Leave on for twenty minutes and remove with warm water.

Oatmeal Dead-Skin Defoliator

1 *cup steel-ground oatmeal*

Pulverize meal in blender and put in large bowl. Bending face over bowl, scoop oatmeal up in handfuls and "wash" your face with the dry meal. Repeat several times; you will end up with a white, floury face, but when you splash warm water to remove the oatmeal residue, you will find the dead layer of cells gone and a wonderfully fresh, rosy skin instead. It's magic.

Honey-Almond Superficial Peeler and Defoliating Mask

3–4 *tablespoons almonds pulverized in blender*
2 *tablespoons honey*

Mix into thick paste and spread onto clean face. Let remain for twenty minutes and remove as if washing your face to allow the abrasiveness of the almonds to remove the dead skin cell layer. Rinse with warm water.

Protein Superficial Peeler and Defoliating Mask

1 *egg yolk*
2 *tablespoons pulverized sea salt*
   (pulverize in blender)

Beat egg yolk until lemon yellow and creamy. Beat in salt. Apply to face and leave on for fifteen minutes. Using the "washing" motion, rub mask gently until it is fully loosened and you can benefit from the abrasiveness of the salt crystals in order to remove dead skin cells. Rinse off with warm water.

Egg-White Beauty Mask
(not for aging skins)

Whip egg white until fluffy. Apply to clean face (oily skins can take several applications, letting each one dry before applying the next) and leave on for twenty minutes. Remove with warm water.

RECIPES FOR BEAUTY MASKS
FOR NORMAL AND DRY SKINS

Wax Pack

2 *tablespoons anhydrous lanolin*
1 *tablespoon beeswax*

Melt together over low heat. Stir together and, when temperature is still warm but cool enough to apply, spread over clean face. Let harden and leave on for fifteen minutes. Peel off, or scrape off gently with a butter knife and rinse face with warm water or remove the residue with a warm, wet washcloth.

Avocado-Butter Mask

¼ *fresh avocado, mashed*
1 *tablespoon margarine*

Warm together over water until warm and spread onto clean face. Leave on for twenty minutes and remove with warm water.

Real Mayonnaise Mask

That's all. Simply spread over clean face and let remain for twenty minutes. Remove with warm water.

Strawberry Clay Mask

3 *tablespoons fuller's earth*
1 *ounce mashed strawberries*
Drop witch hazel

Mix together until thick paste is formed. Spread on clean face and leave for twenty minutes. Remove with warm water. (Pulverized bran or oatmeal can be substituted for Fuller's Earth).

RECIPES FOR BEAUTY MASKS FOR OILY SKIN

Grapefruit Pack

3 *tablespoons fuller's earth (available at*
drugstore)
Grapefruit juice, strained

Mix together until thick paste is formed and spread on clean face. Leave on for twenty minutes and remove with warm water.

Tomato-Oatmeal Mask

¼ *cup steel-ground oatmeal*
(pulverized in blender)
1 *tablespoon dried sage*
Fresh, strained tomato juice

Mix together until thick paste is formed and spread on clean face. Let remain for twenty minutes and remove with warm water.

Cucumber-Mint Mask

> 2 ounces strained cucumber juice
> (pureed in blender)
> 1 tablespoon dried mint
> 1–2 tablespoons whole wheat flour

Mix together into thick paste and spread on clean face. Let remain for twenty minutes and remove with warm water.

Lemon Beauty Mask

> 3 tablespoons pulverized bran
> Juice of one lemon (do not strain)
> Egg white

Mix all together and spread over clean face. Let remain for twenty minutes and remove with warm water.

RECIPES FOR BEAUTY MASKS FOR AGING SKIN

Deep-Penetrating Hot Oil Mask

> ½ cup virgin olive oil
> 1 square cheesecloth

Cut out a mask from cheesecloth to fit face, leaving holes for eyes and mouth. Warm the olive oil and soak cloth in it. Wring out lightly and fit onto clean face. As cloth cools, dip again into warm oil and reapply. Repeat several times. Rinse some of the oil off face with warm water and pat dry, letting the remaining oil continue to penetrate and protect.

Honey-Oatmeal Mask

> ¼ cup steel-ground oatmeal
> (pulverized in blender)
> Honey warmed over water

Mix together into thick paste and spread over clean face. Let remain for twenty minutes and remove with washing motions to help remove dead skin cells. Rinse with warm water.

Butter-Banana Mask

½ *banana, mashed*
1 *tablespoon cocoa butter*

Melt together over low heat, and, when still warm but cool enough to apply, spread over clean face. Leave on for twenty minutes and remove with warm water.

Protein-Wax Pack

1 *egg yolk*
2 *tablespoons anhydrous lanolin*
1 *tablespoon beeswax*

Beat egg yolk until lemon yellow in color and stir into melted lanolin and wax until all ingredients are blended together. When still warm, but cool enough to apply, spread over clean face and let harden for ten to twenty minutes (if your skin is not firm, remove after ten minutes). Peel off gently or remove with butter knife. Rinse face in warm water and remove any residue with a wet, warm washcloth.

Massage Oils

There is almost nothing, repeat *nothing*, as lovely as a homemade massage oil. Most body skin is dry, and therefore can benefit immensely from the penetrating qualities of a good massage oil made from natural vegetable oils. Use these oils not only for professional massages (or personally given massages, to or from your favorite man), but also as after-bath or after-shower moisturizers for the entire body. Especially after a body "facial," you will find your skin feeling smooth as satin and looking just as silky.

Do not put on clothing immediately after the application of these oils; they need around ten minutes to penetrate. Use only small amounts; they are very rich. If you happen to use too much and your body feels too slick, simply towel off the extra oil. Keep all massage oils in the refrigerator between uses to ensure a longer life; few of us are lucky enough to get such a treat every day and use up the entire bottle immediately. You can change the scent by substituting a portion of the oils used with a scented oil or with different flavored extracts.

RECIPES FOR MASSAGE OILS

Almond Massage Oil

4 ounces almond oil
1 ounce liquid lecithin
1 ounce almond extract

Warm oil and stir in lecithin. Heat almond extract and beat into oil (don't worry if it foams) until cool and well blended. Shake before using each time and refrigerate between uses.

Massage Oil for Sore Muscles

4 tablespoons anhydrous lanolin
3 ounces olive oil
1 teaspoon oil of wintergreen
½ teaspoon menthol (may be omitted)

Warm lanolin and olive oil together until blended. Cool. Stir in oil of wintergreen and menthol and put in plastic bottle. (*Do not use on face, and keep away from children.*)

Favorite Perfume Massage Oil

2 ounces sesame oil
½ ounce liquid lecithin
1 ounce favorite cologne

Warm oil and stir in lecithin. Warm perfume only slightly and, dribbling slowly, beat into oil mixture until well blended. Shake before each use.

4

DAILY WAKE-UP WARM-UPS

Don't think of this morning activity as exercise. Think of it as waking up your body . . . for that, in fact, is really all it is. After lying relatively still for eight or so hours, anything needs revitalizing. Have you ever noticed how animals stretch when they first rise up from lying down? Even your car needs warming up in the morning. Humans should warm up and wake up, too.

The most important reasons to *move* each day in some form of mildly vigorous activity are twofold. Number one, your muscles will remain young and strong for a longer period of time if they are stretched regularly. Number two—and most often ignored—physical activity helps to distribute both oxygen and nutrients from your food consumption to the various parts of the body. Not only is digestion improved but circulation as well, both of which are necessary, at any age, for good general health.

Even if you have a serious weight problem (and unless otherwise directed by your doctor), you must move your body in order to promote internal health. You may also find, as many overweight people do, that daily attention paid to your body in the form of some physical activity encourages you to alter your overweight physical appearance as well.

A word should be said here on the relationship of overweight and age.

There is no doubt that *serious* obesity adds years to any appearance, male or female, but this is not primarily a beauty problem; it is a medical problem. If you are more than fifteen or twenty pounds overweight, you are straining your health in a much more detrimental way than you are straining your looks.

On the other hand, in this age of not only youth worship but also "thin" worship, do not fall into the trap of thinking you cannot look younger and lovelier within this ten-day period if you are only ten or even fifteen pounds over what you think you ideally should be. Lose that extra weight or don't lose it—twenty years ago, it wasn't considered "extra." This is an aesthetic decision, not a health danger. A feeling of embarrassment or inferiority about what you consider to be extra weight will do far more to add years (in the way of stress) than the weight itself. You may find, as many do, that when you care for yourself properly in other beauty areas and dress to express your own sense of yourself, the weight problem is much easier to deal with because you feel better about yourself in general.

In any event, extra weight or not, and even if you abhor exercising and have a real urge to skip this part of the program, please do *not* give in to that urge. If you wish to look younger, you must move younger, and the results will be worth it. You will look and feel better.

The following movements do not take long—ten to fifteen minutes tops—but they do prepare both your body and your mind for activity and, over the long run, will do their share in keeping your body toned and alive.

Good Morning Swing

Stand straight with feet comfortably apart and hands on hips. Swing to the count of four: One—hands reaching for the ceiling, straight above head, Two—bend at waist until chest is parallel to the floor, hands outstretched straight in front of your head (keep eyes forward), Three—bend completely forward, hands touch the floor, and Four—stand up straight and return hands to hips. Repeat entire swing sequence six times.

Prancing in Place

Think of this as a pretty jog in place. With hands on hips and head high, prance (pointing toes each time a foot leaves the floor) to the count of one hundred. (If you prefer, jumping rope can be a wonderful alternative to prancing.)

Waist Bends

Stand with feet comfortably apart, arms extended straight above your head with hands clasped. Keeping hands together, bounce three times to the right and three times to the left bending to the side directly at the waist each time. Be sure you lean neither to the front or the back, but *directly* to each side. Repeat to each side six times.

Sit-ups

If you have a weak back, do these sit-ups with your knees bent. Lie on the floor with hands extended above your head. Swing up (it can be helpful to slip your toes under something solid to prevent them from lifting off the floor) and reach hands forward, touching your toes with your hands and trying to touch your head to your knees. On your return trip to the floor, uncurl your body slowly, touching first the small of your back and then each vertebra separately to the floor, keeping shoulders rounded until they, too, touch the floor. Repeat six to ten times.

Knee Bends

Standing with one hand on the back of a chair, place your feet approximately one foot apart. Keeping your *back straight* and your buttocks pulled under, head high and eyes directly to the front, lift your heels slowly off the floor and bend the knees as far as you can go *without* relaxing into the final knee-bend position—you should at all times feel the tension in the tops of your thighs. Return to a standing position by placing the heels on the floor first (while knees are still bent) and then slowly straightening the legs. Repeat six times.

The Fanny Walk

Sit on the floor and bend knees, bringing them up close to your chest. Place hands behind you on the floor to help keep your balance and lift feet off the floor, pointing your toes. Move forward (hands off the floor if you can) on your fanny alone, "scooching" along by moving from one side of the buttocks to the other. The harder you "hit" each side to the floor each time (within reason), the better to break down the fat deposits in the overly padded derriere almost all women have managed to acquire.

Posture Set

Stand straight, pull waist up and out of hips, pull buttocks under. Raise shoulders and try to touch your ears. Keeping shoulders high, round them forward as far as you can go; now (still keeping them high) press them back as far as they will go; and finally drop them back into place to properly align your posture. (It can be helpful to repeat this short procedure from time to time throughout the day. One of the great agers is poor posture.)

Special Attention to Trouble Spots

FOR THE ABDOMEN

Leg Raises

Lie flat on the floor, making sure the small of your back is pressing into the floor. Bend knees and raise them toward chest. Straighten legs until they are straight up at a right angle to your body and perpendicular to the floor. *Slowly* lower legs back toward the floor, stopping when feet are still two or three inches from the floor. Bend knees to the chest again (this is the point at which to rest if you need to) and repeat. If you find this exercise too strenuous at the beginning, do one leg at a time. Should be repeated eight times.

Curl-ups

Lie flat on the floor, making sure the small of your back is touching the floor. Bend both knees, keeping feet flat on the floor. Curl your head and upper body upward into a forty-five-degree angle (do not straighten your body) and hold to the count of six. Slowly reverse the movement until you are again lying flat on the floor. Repeat eight times.

"V" Hold

Sit on the floor with your legs spread apart in front of you. Cup the right hand backward into the instep of the right foot (bending the knee to grasp the foot) and straighten the leg up and to the right side. Still holding the right leg in that position, repeat the procedure with the left leg. You will now be seated on your buttocks alone with both hands holding both legs up and to the sides to form a "V." Tighten your stomach muscles and hold in this position to the count of six, relax and repeat eight times. (If you have difficulty holding your balance in the beginning, do one leg at a time until you can straighten the leg easily, and then practice holding your balance. In order to practice balance, you may lift both legs simultaneously just to get the feeling, but eventually you should extend one leg at a time and then hold for the count.) This is also good for the hamstring muscles at the back of your thighs.

FOR THE THIGHS AND HIPS

Three-Position Kicks

Lie on your side, leaning your body on one arm bent at the elbow. Place the other hand flat on the floor, elbow bent, in front of you. Now, roll slightly *back* on your hip and raise and lower the top leg swiftly, to the side and slightly front, ten times. Next (without resting the leg on the floor), roll *forward* on your hip until you are just midway and can lift your leg directly up to the side. Repeat leg lifts ten times. Lastly, roll *forward further* on hip so that your leg lifts will be slightly to the back, and repeat ten more swift lifts. Roll over to the other side and repeat entire exercise.

Table Kicks

Kneel on both knees, placing both hands (with the elbows straight) on the floor in front of you, putting your back parallel to the ceiling. You should be now more or less in the shape of a table. Lift head and look in front of you. Raise one knee up and to the side, so that your knee is nearly touching your elbow. Alternately straighten and bend leg twenty times. Repeat with other leg.

Leg Scissors

Lie flat on your back, making sure the small of your back is touching the floor. Bring knees up to your chest. Open legs, stretch and straighten them to the sides in the form of open scissors. Now, bring them together over your body (closing the scissors) and cross them, smacking your inner thighs together as you do so. Open them again and repeat the procedure twenty times.

FOR THE BUTTOCKS

Belly Dancing Hip Circles

Stand with feet approximately two feet apart and knees bent slightly. Hold arms out (at about breast height) with elbows slightly bent, palms facing front. Contract both buttocks muscles tightly and, moving only the hip and buttock area, make a complete circle to the right. When the hips are facing front again, repeat the motion to the left. Each time you complete half the circle (to the back), release the buttock muscles, and then tighten them again as you continue the circle to the front. Repeat both directions ten times.

Belly Dancing Hip Stops

This is similar to the above except that you move the hips swiftly from position to position. Stand as directed above, but instead of circling slowly to the right, thrust the right hip into a locked position, tightening the *right* buttock and the right thigh at the same time. (This exercise has a "striptease" quality to it.) Next, thrust both buttocks to the back and release all muscles. Then thrust *left* hip into a locked position, tightening the muscles in the left buttock and the left thigh, and finally, lift both hips to the front (a real "bump"), tightening both buttocks. Instead of the previous slow circle, you are here thrusting the hips into four "stopped" positions—right, back, left, front—that form a square. Repeat in both directions ten times.

FOR THE MIDRIFF

Arm Stretches

Stand facing front with feet approximately two feet apart. Reach for the ceiling with your left hand, and, bending the waist to the right side, lean the entire upper torso to the right, keeping the hand over your head. Now, *push* that hand (fingers pointed to the right) farther to the right (your entire arm is over your head parallel to the ceiling), using the whole arm as you bounce the upper torso to the right. You should feel the muscles pull through your *left* midriff section. Bounce two times and then bend farther, as far to the right as you can, and s-t-r-e-t-c-h the arm, pushing it toward the right wall, pulling those left muscles taut. Repeat sequence eight times. Repeat exercise to the left, extending the right arm.

Arm Twists

Stand as directed above. With your right hand, grasp the four raised fingers of your left hand. Next, *twist* your entire upper torso to the right and back and, with your right hand, *pull* the left arm toward the back wall. You should feel the muscles in the *back* of the left midriff section being pulled. Pull eight times and repeat exercise to the other side. Repeat in both directions eight times.

Arm Reaches

Stand as directed above. Raise both arms above your head straight up and as far apart as your shoulders. Now, alternately *reach* for the ceiling with each hand, stretching the right midriff section when you reach with your right hand and vice versa. Repeat each hand reach ten times. This exercise also helps firm upper arms.

FOR THE UPPER ARMS

Arm Circles

Stand facing front with feet approximately two feet apart. Stretch arms to each side, letting elbows bend *only slightly*. Make tiny circles with your hands toward the front wall twenty times. Reverse direction and repeat toward the back wall. You should feel the strain in the upper portions of both arms.

As a variation, stand as directed above, but bend elbows farther and turn the palms of both hands toward the front wall. Now, raise both shoulders toward your ears and make a half-circle to the front with your hands (keeping the palms facing forward), bringing the shoulders into a forward "shrugged" position at the same time. Circle arms up and return to starting position. Now, raise shoulders up and half-circle the hands to the back, thrusting shoulders back and down as well. Return to starting position. You should feel the pull in both upper arms and in the backs of each shoulder. Repeat entire procedure eight times.

(The above exercises are also beneficial in firming the breast area.)

FOR THE BREASTS (TO FIRM)

Arm Pushes

Bend arms in front of you (Indian-style), with each hand grasping the forearm of the opposite arm. Now, *push* each forearm toward the elbow and release pressure. Repeat movement once each second in a continuous succession of little pushes. You will feel little *pulls* in both breasts. Give twenty to thirty pushes before stopping.

Rowing Pulls

Stand with feet approximately two feet apart and stretch arms to each side. Bring both arms to the front until they are parallel to each other and then, closing hands into fists, pull elbows directly back until fists are directly at the side of each breast and elbows are pulled back and up as far as they will go (this is like the exaggerated motion of rowing a boat). Repeat exercise ten times.

5

MAKING UP, NOT OVER

I do not believe in making "over." It may be true that a certain color or hairstyle or eye-makeup combination might be, objectively, most flattering to your individual features, but if it doesn't also express the inner you—the only real individuality you have—and suit your own particular life-style, then I would not recommend it. When it comes to makeup in particular, make-overs almost never work in the long run. I also have erred in the past, giving a woman a magnificent "new" face only to see her a week later wearing the same "old" one because she feels the new techniques aren't really *her*.

Therefore, in this chapter, I will outline the principles of applying makeup. Once you understand these, you can adapt your own face to any fad or fashion that may come—and go—if you choose to; or you can find the one, simple method for very naturally enhancing what you already have without making any drastic changes. The first is rather like redecorating a whole room from top to bottom; the second, more like putting a fresh coat of paint on a room you're already very happy with— it won't necessarily look "different," but it will certainly look newer (younger), fresher (younger) and brighter (younger).

The Principles of Makeup

The purpose of normal, everyday makeup is *not* to create an image or to re-create your face. It *is* to help you look like yourself . . . your best and youngest self. Knowledgeable application of makeup can emphasize those aspects of your features that are most pleasing (to yourself and others) and detract from less important or less attractive aspects.

Makeup can be used to add startling, dramatic or fun elements for dramatic or fun occasions, but, for general use, it should be used for brightening and finishing (and youthening) your own natural assets and personality. You may find it helpful to take notes in chapter 13's "Work Sheets" as you go through this chapter in order to specifically note suggestions that you don't want to forget.

A few overall hints may prove useful at the start:

1. Never apply makeup *directly* to any wrinkled area. It only increases the depth of the wrinkles by collecting in them as well as drawing attention to that area.

2. Never press powder into any lined area for the same reason as above. Use only a brush and loose powder as instructed later in this chapter.

3. For a youthful effect, remember that the less product you use the better. Not a lesser *number* of products, but less of the *amount* of each product. A "small amount" and "blend well" are good watchwords. (Don't be intimidated by this warning and use so little it achieves no effect; just watch out for that overly made-up look that adds years to anyone.)

4. Keep your face moist throughout the day by (tapping with your fingertips) patting a small amount of moisturizer or petroleum jelly over any especially dry areas (right over makeup) to maintain a dewy, young appearance throughout the day.

5. Once you have finished applying whichever makeup look you wish, blushes of pink can help to create a youthful effect regardless of your basic color scheme. Instructions are given later in this chapter.

6. Don't be afraid to experiment or move your products around. There is nothing wrong with using lipstick as a blusher or using eye shadow on your cheeks. Blushers make excellent lip liners, etc., so try to permit your mind a great deal of flexibility concerning the whole subject of makeup. Foundations can be mixed, as can nail enamels. If you unfetter your imagination, you'll soon see how many different products can be moved around the face with surprisingly happy results.

7. In order to youthen any face with makeup, keep the colors soft. This does not mean using pale colors, but subtle colors—no bright or harsh reds, or purples or oranges on lips and cheeks; no stark blues or greens around the eyes.

8. Frosted makeup of any kind is *out* during the day if you wish to look younger, unless you want (and can carry off) a very dramatic statement.

9. Do not rely on color makeup computers, offered by some cosmetic houses, to select your makeup schemes. At best, they will prevent you from making drastic mistakes in the realm of color choices, but they can never offer you the individualized aspects of makeup selection that is the key to enhancing your own very individual face.

The Application of Makeup

UNDEREYE CONCEALER—MAGIC TRICK NUMBER ONE

There is no magic in makeup, any more than in anything else, of course, but certain little tricks have such an immediate, youthful effect on appearance that they seem to be magical. The correct application of undereye concealer is one of those tricks. The purpose of this product is to lighten the area directly under the eyes, where discoloration and bagginess have a tendency to appear. It is the first product to be applied in any complete makeup application.

Undereye concealer comes in both pot and stick forms. I recommend the pot form because the skin under the eye is very thin and delicate; application via a stick usually results in pushing and pulling the skin too roughly. This product—in whatever form you choose to purchase it— should be applied with the little finger for two reasons: One, it is the smallest and can get into narrow portions of the areas to be covered; and two, most people usually exert less pressure on the skin when using the least strong finger.

Color of Undereye Concealer

Select a neutral, beige or ivory color that is *slightly* lighter than your natural skin tone. If you choose a depth of color that is too light, it will give the appearance of "clown white" under your eyes and, rather than detracting from any discoloration or tiredness there, will bring attention to the area instead. If you have deep discoloration, *pink* undereye concealer can be very helpful (be sure to blend a bit of foundation over it).

Texture of Undereye Concealer

This is most important. Undereye concealer should be creamy smooth and go on easily. Any product that is dry or sticky at all will increase the depth of any lines you may have already acquired, and it will dry out the skin and give you a caked, made-up appearance.

Application of Undereye Concealer

Using the little finger, apply the product a little at a time with a light "tapping" motion. Do not rub this delicate area. "Tap" and "blend" are the watchwords here. Later, you will use the same method to blend your foundation into and over the concealer. Only a little product is needed; do not attempt to cover completely. Don't forget, you are after an overall effect, and undereye concealer is only one of the several methods to be utilized. Apply the product in an "L" shape according to the illustration below. Do not apply *directly* to laugh lines. Blend into that area for a uniform look. (See illustration: Arrows indicate direction of tap-tap blending of undereye concealer out and into the rest of the face.)

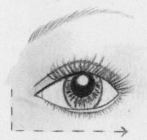

Placement of undereye concealer

FOUNDATION

The purpose of foundation is to even out the natural color of your facial skin. It may help to think of its application as similar to the preparation of a canvas for painting. Like an artist, you need uniformity of texture and color as a background before beginning to shape the subject. In this case, the subject is the sum of your own features.

First, examine and determine the natural, overall color tone of your skin. Is it ruddy (reddish)? Or sallow (yellow)? Or olive (slightly green)? Or creamy without any tinge of the above?

Color of Foundation

The best method of "cleaning the canvas" is to apply a light coat of neutralizer before you apply a completely neutral shade of foundation.

Not all cosmetic companies offer this product, and the ones who do give different names to these neutralizers; if not "neutralizer" itself, you may find it by asking for an under-foundation "toner."

Neutralizers come in five basic colors: pink or rose, coral, green, lavender and blue. If your skin is *very ruddy*, use green. If only *slightly ruddy*, use lavender. If your skin is *sallow*, use pink or rose. If it is *olive*, use pink or coral, depending on the particular shade of greenish tint your natural skin seems to carry. Only if you have a *ruddy* or a *creamy* complexion can you use blue, which gives a transluscent, porcelain quality (best saved for evening wear) to the finished look.

You must experiment with these neutralizers in a department store before you purchase any one product. Remove all makeup except undereye concealer and eye makeup. Cream your face and *lightly* apply the color you think best (do not apply *over* undereye concealer). Next, apply a neutral shade of foundation. Examine the color tone of your skin (in daylight) at this point. It should look absolutely bland in color but carry a definite quality of "aliveness." It should not appear "covered," merely like a naturally even and uniformly colored, healthy, glowing skin tone.

Foundation is not a product with which you should add color to your skin; this is achieved with other products. The use of neutralizers and foundations is strictly to give the skin a clarity, a uniformity and a neutrality in color tone.

However . . . as a reluctant alternative to my last thought, I will offer another method of foundation selection to any "lazies" who will refuse to take the time to carry out my best recommendation. This is, at least, better than nothing. If your skin is *ruddy*, choose a completely neutral shade of foundation: beige; no hints of rose or coral whatsoever. If your skin is *sallow*, select a shade with a slight hint of rose. If it is *olive*, a drop of coral or pink in the color will enliven the natural skin tone. If your skin is creamy and evenly colored already, the sheerest neutral shade you can find will give a finished, polished appearance. I repeat, this method of foundation selection is not even second best, it is fifth best; but it is better than nothing.

Depth of Foundation Shade

In selecting the depth of any foundation shade itself, apply a few drops directly to your neck area. You will, of course, be selecting a lighter shade if your skin is pale and a deeper shade if your skin tone is darker, but the foundation should closely match the skin tone of your neck.

If you cannot find one that matches exactly, select a shade *slightly* darker than your own skin. Never lighter—it gives a masklike appearance.

Consistency, or Texture, of Foundation

First, if you have a dry or normal skin, you should use an *oil-based* foundation. If you have an oily skin, you should use a *water-based* foundation. If you have a combination skin (part oily and part dry), you will have to experiment to see which one feels best, depending on the amount and distribution of the natural oils in your own particular combination.

Once you have decided the above, you must decide what kind of "coverage" you need. Not to achieve a covered look, but merely to help you achieve the surface clarity discussed earlier. If you have a clear complexion with no eruptions or brown spots, the sheerest texture you can find in a foundation would be best. If you do have any distracting surface imperfections, try a foundation with a little heavier texture in order to even out the surface of your skin as well as the color. Be careful never to use a too heavily textured foundation; it can collect in any wrinkled areas and add age rather than detract from it.

Your foundation might be a good place to begin individualizing your beauty products and losing your fears of mixing and matching. If you already have some old foundations, try mixing some of them together to achieve the correct color you now desire before you run out and buy a new one. If you have the right color, but not the right texture, add a little mineral oil or moisturizing lotion if it is too drying or some water if it is too thick. You must learn to adapt beauty products to suit your needs.

Don't forget the main purposes of a foundation. One: It should neutralize and unify the natural *color* of your skin. Two: It should retain the natural *depth* of color you have in your own skin. Three: It should contribute to the clarity of your natural skin by covering any surface imperfections, thereby achieving a smooth appearance. Foundation should, in the end, help you achieve a finished, subtly polished, healthy but bland appearance to your facial skin.

Method of Application

When applying, be sure to blend your foundation down into the neck area to avoid a masked look, slightly and subtly into the hairline and over your ears if your hair is short.

There is no "right" way to apply foundation. If you need very little coverage, a little smoothed on the center of the forehead, the nose and the chin and neck could be enough, merely blending into, not covering completely, the natural skin at the sides of your face. If full coverage is needed, you can pour a little into the palm of one hand, rub your hands together and smooth your hands lightly all over your face, blending as you go. If you prefer to go more slowly, put a few drops on the forehead, blend, then a few drops on the cheeks, blend, next a fair amount on the neck and blend up over the chin and last, a drop or two on the nose blending out to the cheek area. Always tap and blend upward to merge your foundation slightly into your undereye concealer (not cover it) so there are no lines of demarcation. You may wish to moisten a small sponge and apply your foundation with that instead of your fingers. Whatever method seems easy and natural for you should be employed. It's the finished look that matters; how you achieve it is up to you.

CONTOURING—MAGIC TRICK NUMBER TWO

Unless you have a perfectly proportioned face, contouring can become your best friend. Like undereye concealer, it seems to work miracles in erasing age.

The principle to remember here is that dark colors diminish (detract) and light colors highlight (attract). Some cosmetic companies offer specific products for these two purposes, but the results can be accomplished perfectly well by using a medium-brown eyeshadow (or dark foundation or brown blusher) and your undereye concealer (or ivory eyeshadow). Contouring is done *after* your application of foundation is completed but *before* you add color to your face.

Following is a list of contouring tricks to suit your every need. Pick and choose according to your own requirements. Apply the brown shadow sparingly and blend well; contouring must not "show." You must work carefully in order to achieve this miracle. Otherwise, as I caution my lecture audiences, "You will look as if you've been cleaning the fireplace." Use a brush, a damp sponge or your fingers, whatever works best for you. Use cream or dry eyeshadow, whichever you prefer or your skin type dictates—cream on dry skin and powder on oily skin. Don't be afraid of contouring, just be subtle. The results are well worth the effort. Remember only this: Use brown on anything you want to diminish and ivory on anything you want to bring forward.

Brown
1. To create cheekbones and give definition to a round or heavy face:

Blend just under natural cheekbones (suck in the sides of your face, pursing your lips to define the cheekbones) from the center of each cheek up and into the hairline. Don't worry if it looks strange at this point; once blusher is applied and blended into it, the obvious line of the shadow that you see now will disappear into the wonderful illusion of a hollowed facial structure.

2. To slim a round face:
Blend along each side of the face, blending carefully into the hairline.

3. To slim a full jawline or diminish a double chin:
Blend along the edge of the jaw and down into the neck below the chin.

4. To shorten a high forehead:
Blend from the center of the hairline down to the center of the forehead and back up to the hairline in a *wide* "V."

5. To soften a square forehead or chin:
Blend downward or upward from the corners of the "square" just beyond the spot where a normal oval would occur.

6. To slim a large nose:
Blend down both sides of the nose. (You can create an even slimmer effect by blending ivory between the two streaks of brown.)

7. To straighten a crooked nose:
Blend brown into the outer curve and ivory into the inner curve of the bend.

8. To shorten a long nose:
Blend onto the tip of the nose.

Ivory

1. To "lift" cheekbones and add emphasis to eyes:
Blend a thin line along the very top of each cheekbone, above blusher.

2. To bring forward a receding chin:
Blend into bottom and center of chin.

3. To widen a narrow forehead:
Blend into temples and up onto each side of forehead.

4. To heighten a low forehead:
Blend from center of forehead up and into hairline in a wide "V."

5. To widen a narrow face:

Blend along the side of the face—from the eyes down to the jawline—and into the hairline.

6. To camouflage discoloration of eyelids:
   Cover area evenly *before* applying eye makeup.
7. To widen a narrow nose:
   Blend down both sides of nose.
8. To lengthen a short nose:
   Blend a narrow line down center of nose including tip and blend small strips of brown on either side.
9. To soften shadows created by lines (corners of mouth or lines from the nose to the mouth especially):
   Blend into the inner side of the line where the shadow is cast.
10. To create even more highly defined cheekbones:
    Blend into area of face *between* the dark contouring along the jawbone and that under the cheekbone.

Coloring Your Face

It is very advantageous to decide on a basic color palette for your face. This means that whatever daily color scheme you select, it will always reflect the one underlying "color tone" you have chosen to individualize to your face. This can be an important method of personalizing your own makeup style, because it establishes a continuity to your overall look and suggests a prevailing breath of life that becomes your very own. It consists of touching (highlighting) your face in some way with the same color every day regardless of whatever other effects you may achieve.

Brunettes with olive skin usually look best with added rose, plum or mauve color touches.

Brunettes with sallow skin will usually find pink best.

Redheads look marvelous in bronze or peach or even more stunning in mauve or plum, depending upon their skin tone.

Blondes usually look best in bronze, peach, gold or mauve. This may at first sound obvious or conventional, but the truth is that to add pink as a palette color to a blonde usually makes her look too "fluffy" and any of the other palettes are simply to strong.

In practice, utilizing a basic color palette means, first, selecting the rest of your makeup colors to harmonize with your basic color. For example, if your basic palette color is bronze, you would generally select brown eyeliner rather than gray, since brown more easily harmonizes with bronze. Then, at the finish of your completed makeup, each day, you simply "touch" your face (which mean literally touch-tapping with a finger or two) and blend your palette color into the following places: somewhere on your forehead (could be the top-center or top-sides or just above the eyes, depending on which area you would like to subtly highlight), somewhere on your cheeks (usually at the very top of your blusher or just in front of the hairline, blending well), somewhere on your chin (usually the center, unless it is prominent), on your nose (at the tip or subtly down the center) or possibly on the beginning of the cheek area just to either side of the nose and just beneath your undereye concealer. Touching your completed eye makeup (generally at the outer edge) can also be most compelling.

Remember, touching your face with your basic color is done at the very end of your makeup. I mention it here only because you must select this basic color before you choose other, accompanying colors, in order to maintain harmony throughout all of your makeup.

Generally speaking, as far as depth of shade is concerned, a rose, plum or mauve palette can carry stronger accompanying colors if used on a brunette with dark skin. Mauves and pinks on a sallow brunette will call for accompanying products in medium shades, and fair-skinned brunettes will do best with a paler palette (though not as pale as a blonde's). Redheads can select any depth of shade, depending on the strength of their hair color and the tone of their complexion. Blondes will generally find their most attractive look with a soft palette, although dark eyes allow a blonde to do most anything (my own personal palette, for example, is cinnamon).

The best method of discovering your own palette color is to experiment with several different lipstick or blusher colors and shades on a freshly "cleaned canvas" (a face wearing only foundation), touching your face in the above-mentioned places to see which color tone best brings your face to life. You will have to start fresh each time you experiment because there is no way to remove the color without removing the foundation as well. Be patient. This can be an important part of your total look. If you are willing to delay your decision, simply try a different palette color at the end of your makeup each day for a week or so. You'll find the one you like.

EYE MAKEUP

Your eyes are without doubt the most important feature of your face. Of anyone's face. Even if you have a stunningly shaped mouth or a cute nose, it is from your eyes that other people learn most about you. Therefore, makeup emphasis is very important here. If you use too little, you will lose the benefit of emphasis, but if you use too much, the makeup will distract a viewer from the meanings in your eyes themselves. It has been my observation that most women who wear eye makeup wear too much. The most common mistakes are using too-obvious eyeliner or creating bright patches of either blue or green above each eye. Eye makeup should be subtle for everyday wear.

The basic principles are very simple; however, since eyes come in all sizes and shapes, you will have to experiment a bit to discover precisely what is best for you. The principle of light-highlighting and dark-diminishing applies here as well as in face contouring, so remember it when you adapt the following instructions to your own eyes.

Eyeshadow

Color should be selected to emphasize, *not* match, the color of your eyes (nothing is as boring as to see blue eyeshadow on blue eyes) *or* to blend with or accent the color scheme of any particular day's clothing. The latter is far more interesting because the variety is greater; as you vary your clothing choices, so you can also vary your makeup. Any color eye can wear any color eyeshadow if you keep it subtle. You can always tie the unity of your look back together again by touching your finished eye with your basic palette color.

The depth of the color of your eyes is very important, however. If you have pale eyes, the shades and hues of your selections should be more subtle—mauve, not purple; gray-blue, not blue; celery, not grass green; peach, not coral; etc. Bright primary colors will only overpower the eyes themselves. Dark eyes can use stronger shades, but subtle hues of color are recommended for all eye colors. I emphasize this because lack of subtlety creates a blotchy look. It is the eyes that should stand out— not the eye makeup.

TEXTURE OF EYESHADOW

Certainly the texture of eyeshadow is an optional choice. However, if you have any sort of wrinkled (or crepey) appearance above the eye, I would recommend cream eyeshadows because they will not further dry out the area and deepen creases. If cream shadow seems to find its way into the creases, you can simply press a finger to the area and it will smooth out again.

Powder or pressed eyeshadows last longer on the eye, however; so, unless you have the above problem, they can look fresher longer. Even these dry shadows can "run" because the temperature of the eyelid is higher than that of other parts of the face, and this factor alone can melt any makeup, causing problems. If melting eye makeup is a problem for you, there are products on the market called eye makeup bases, which go on under any other eye makeup and which work rather well.

APPLICATION OF EYESHADOW

Whatever the color or depth or shape of your eyes, you will need *three* shades of eye shadow. They can be different shades of the same color or two or three different harmonizing colors. You will need:

—a medium shade for the eyelid
—a light shade for under the eyebrow
—a deeper shade for the eye bone

The eyelid color sets your basic color scheme. Remember that light color brings forward and deeper color recedes a feature, so if your eyes protrude at the eyelid, you will want to choose a medium shade on the deeper side to set them back. If your eyes are deeply set, you will need a medium shade on the lighter side to bring them forward. Bring this medium color up and over the brow bone but not up as far as the eyebrow. Next, apply the palest shade under the eyebrow. (See illustration.)

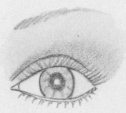

Medium and light shades of eyeshadow

It is with the deepest shade of eyeshadow that you create the "shadow" or any real effect you wish. Here, you must experiment on your own eyes. Most eyes will look best with the deep shade approximately in the middle of the other two, contrasting shades—following the natural line just under and blended up onto the brow bone slightly (if the bone above your eye is not apparent, find it with your finger). It is with this deep shade that you contour the eye and create depth. Depending on the shape of your eye, your deep shade could be used just to form a crease of a shadow, or perhaps your eye will look larger and brighter if you pull the color up almost to the eyebrow on the outside. Or you could create a crease with the deep shade and carry it to the outer edge of your eye and then bring another line of the same color out from under your eye to meet it creating a horizontal V around the eyes (see illustrations). I could give you illustrations of a dozen different eye shapes and indicate precisely the spot for this shadowing shade, but *your* eye would still probably not be illustrated. Everyone's eyes are shaped differently. The only way to find the best combination of these three shades is to experiment. Each day of this program, try just a little different placement of this deeper shade (within the basic, indicated areas, of course) and see the different effects you can achieve. Note: If your eyes are very deep-set you may achieve a more flattering effect by eliminating this deep shade altogether, using only medium and light shades and blending them well.

Eyeshadow may be applied with Q-tips, sponges, brushes or your fingers—but the *final* blending must be done with fingers or a brush in order to achieve a subtle, blended effect.

Eyeliner
Eyeliner comes in a variety of applicators. Any and all of them are quite acceptable (pencils, cakes, tubes), but if you select the liquid type that

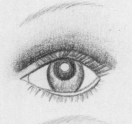

Deeper shade of eyeshadow crease

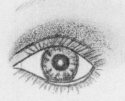

Deeper shade of eyeshadow over eyebrow bone

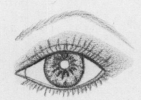

Deeper shade of eyeshadow in horizontal V

comes with its own brush, do *not* use the brush provided (it is almost always too large). To apply any cake or liquid liner, it is best to purchase a very fine, natural-bristled artist's brush from an art store or a fine brush (more expensive) especially designed for eyeliner at your cosmetic counter.

Eyeliner can be used for a variety of purposes.

To thicken the appearance of your lashes and emphasize the eyes themselves—select brown, black, gray, taupe or plum, depending upon the color of your eyes, the depth of their shade or your eyeshadow color scheme. (Very stark, dark colors do not usually look well on pale eyes unless the lashes are naturally dark to begin with. Dark colors also tend to make already small eyes smaller.) Next, line the upper and one-half to three-quarters of the lower lashes by one of three methods.

1. Apply dots very close together along the edge and in between lashes for a natural look—best done with a brush.

2. Lay a brush sideways along the root of the lashes (this is especially helpful if your hand is not too steady), dragging it slowly along until entire lash is lined.

3. "Paint" the line on, using the brush as it was intended, or "pencil" it on if that is what you prefer.

To smudge or not is up to you. The line can be left defined for a

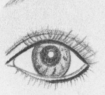

Eyeliner to thicken lashes and emphasize eyes

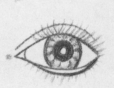

Eyeliner to widen eyes

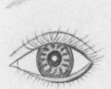

Eyeliner to brighten color of eyes

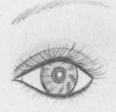

Eyeliner to make eyes appear smaller or create evening drama with lashes

more sophisticated, made-up look or smudged with your finger or a cotton swab for a more natural smoky look. Do not be intimidated by the latest fashion in eyeliners; whatever looks best on your eyes is what's best for you. Some eyes can go without eyeliner altogether.

To widen an eye, apply white eyeliner pencil *inside* the bottom lash (on that little ledge you will find if you gently pull the eye down) before you add other, darker liner. A tiny point of red blusher dotted on with a brush and pressed once with a fingertip to smudge it—at the very inside corner of the eye, not inside the eye itself—can brighten this effect as well.

To brighten the color of your eyes (by making the white of the eye look whiter), apply dark blue eyeliner pencil inside the ledge of the bottom lash as described above. You can also use the same blue pencil, lining under the bottom lash to heighten the effect, and, if you wish, lift the top lash and line the underside of the top lid as well.

To create the illusion of a smaller eye (especially good if eyes protrude), line the inside ledge of both the upper and lower lashes with brown or dark gray, depending upon the lightness or darkness of your natural lash color. This "closes" the eye somewhat. In the evening, especially if artificial lashes are used to open the eyes back up again, this method of lining can create a dramatic effect for anyone. (See illustrations on facing page.)

Mascara

The purpose of mascara is to lengthen and thicken your natural lashes. It can be applied with a brush in either liquid or cake form, whichever you prefer.

The natural color of your own eyelashes (not your eyes) determines the color of mascara you should use. If your natural lashes are pale, black mascara usually gives an artificial appearance; soft brown or gray would give a subtler effect. Dark lashes, of course, can take the deepest shade of brown, charcoal or black. Dark lashes *and* dark eyes will obtain their greatest advantage from black (midnight blue can also have a stunning effect upon this combination).

Apply mascara by first lowering the eyelid and brushing a small quantity down onto the upper side of the tips of the lashes. Next, with the eye wide open, brush mascara on horizontally from the outside of the eyelash toward the inside corner. Last, brush upward, separating and placing the lashes in their final upward curl. On bottom lashes, brush horizontally in both directions until the desired effect is achieved.

If you wish a thicker appearance, let the first coat of mascara dry, fluff a brush of powder over the lashes and add another application of mascara.

(You may or may not choose to use an eyelash curler. They are wonderfully effective and I recommend them highly, but if your natural lashes are already curled, there is no need for one; or if your own lashes are sparse and come out easily, it would be ill advised. If you have never used a curler before, they are available in the dime store and directions are right on the package.)

Artificial Eyelashes

Unless you have the time and patience to apply them individually, one at a time, these almost never look attractive during the day. However, if you wish to wear "strip" lashes, day or night, they must be applied properly in order to look natural. The most important principle here is to make sure that the last lash "showing," at either end of the eye, is your own eyelash. In other words, cut the artificial lash a little bit on each end until it is not apparent at either end when placed above your own lashes; the artificial lash should never overextend your own lashes. The length and thickness of the artificial lash should also be trimmed with a small manicuring scissors or a razor blade until it gives the appearance of merely thickening and slightly lengthening your own lashes. Artificial eyelashes should not show. If they do, they detract from your eyes rather than enhance them.

Eyebrows

Since your eyebrows frame your eyes, I consider them part of your eye makeup.

The eyebrow issue is a bit tricky. Generally speaking, it is best to accept the judgment of Mother Nature and avoid any drastic change in the placement or the natural line of your eyebrows. If you do, by plucking them too thin and penciling them to death, the result is usually one not only of added years, but also of extremely unattractive artificiality. Remember, anything that attracts attention to itself and away from your eyes defeats its purpose.

The area between the eyes should be cleaned completely of stray hairs, of course, leaving the beginning edge of the brows above approximately the same points as the inner corners of your eyes. Using a pencil, create a vertical line alongside your nose and past the inner corner of your eye. The point where the pencil neets your eyebrow is generally (give or take a little, according to your own physiognomy) the place where your brows should begin. Taking the same pencil, create another line from the bottom of the nose past the outside corner of your eye. The point where the pencil meets the outer edge of your natural brow is generally the point to which you should shorten or, with pencil, extend the brow. (See illustration.)

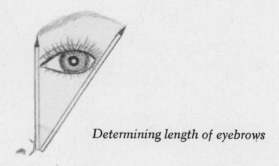

Determining length of eyebrows

If your eyebrow seems to "crowd" your eye from above, you can open up the space between the eye and the lower line of the brow by removing hairs beneath the brow, leaving the shape of the arch the same or lifting it only slightly—a too severely arched brow looks as artificial as a too plucked brow. The finished brow should have a tamed, neat appearance; any tangled or straggly hairs should be removed. It has been my observation that the most common error in eyebrows is overshaping. Unless you have a facial structure as flawless as Garbo's, leave the penciled look alone.

In order to fill in or further shape your brows, use short, feathered strokes with a fine pencil to finish your look. Use a color one shade lighter than your natural brow color.

Very dark eyebrows should be lightened with a bleach to one shade lighter than the color of your hair (unless your hair is blond, and then the brows should be one shade darker). Note: If you use a tint or bleach on your eyebrows, apply it carefully and sparingly. Sit still and observe your eyes every minute of the time the dye is on your brows (usually five minutes is enough) to avoid any of it dripping into your eyes. This could be serious and even cause blindness, so if you choose to lighten or tint your eyebrows, *be careful*. Wipe the bleach off carefully and completely when you are finished and carefully wash the area with soap and water.

LIPSTICK

Apply it any way you like—with your fingers, from pots, tubes, brushes, sticks, wands—but definition of the lip line can be achieved only with a lip brush or pencil.

Lips should be outlined for two main purposes: to *slightly* change the shape of the lips if that is desired, or to maintain at least some outline color on the lips when your lipstick wears off.

If your purpose is the latter, merely use a lip brush to line the edges of your lips with whatever normal lipstick you are using to fill in the rest of your lips. Then, later in the day, as your lip color wanes, you will still have some definition left outlining the lips' shape until you refresh your lipstick.

If you wish to slightly alter the lips' natural lines, try the following (and see illustrations on next page):

• To "pout" your lip appearance a bit, outline your normal lip line and the sides of the lips themselves with a color darker than the one with which you fill in the center.
• To enlarge your lips, outline either the lower or upper (or both) slightly—please *only* slightly—above or below the normal lip line.
• To make your lips appear smaller, outline either the lower or upper (or both) slightly inside the normal lip line.
• To narrow an entire mouth that is too wide, add a little drop of a darker color to the center of your lips.

If your lips are really exceptionally large and actually oversized for your face, you can sometimes cover them completely with under-eye concealer or foundation and then carefully "paint" on a smaller lip. This takes practice and a steady hand, but it can work. I recommend it, however, only if you have a serious size problem, because it can tend to look artificial if not done artfully.

I recommend lip gloss only on the full lip area of the mouth. If you outline the lips with it, it tends to make the color run, especially if you have any small wrinkle lines around the mouth area. (If you have such wrinkles, line your lips with either a pencil or noncreamy lipstick and avoid dark colors.)

As far as lip color is concerned, the biggest mistake many women make is selecting a color that is too bright or too dark. This is almost always harsh and unattractive *and* aging, especially so if there is any

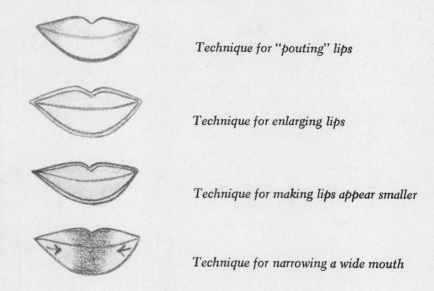

Technique for "pouting" lips

Technique for enlarging lips

Technique for making lips appear smaller

Technique for narrowing a wide mouth

yellow cast to the teeth. Lip color should never overpower eye makeup in depth or intensity; otherwise it will detract from everyone's most important feature—the inner self, as expressed in the eyes. Remember your basic palette color when selecting lip color to ensure harmony and then select a light (not pale) or medium shade compatible with the depth of color you wear on your eyes and cheeks. These three makeup centers —eyes, cheeks and lips—should be balanced for depth of shade. The only exception to this rule is if you wish to emphasize your eyes; then you would keep your mouth and cheek colors slightly lighter in order to throw attention to the eyes.

CHEEK MAKEUP

Once again, your basic color palette should be kept in mind when selecting cheek color. You may vary it daily according to the color of any clothing you may happen to be wearing, but the color should always harmonize with your palette color.

If you have dry skin, select a cream blusher. If you have oily skin, choose dry cheek color and apply with a soft brush.

The placement of cheek color is important. A general rule to remember: Confine the color to the upper half of your face, above the tip of your nose. Since our purpose is to create a youthful effect throughout, I am recommending a horizontal "V" placement of cheek color to give life to the entire upper portion of the face, thereby "lifting" the general appearance. (See illustration below.)

Blend well into the hairline so that no lines of demarcation are apparent and, after smoothing the color on, tap and blend further into place with your fingers to achieve a completely natural look. If you have contoured your cheekbones, blend the cheek color into and slightly over the brown shadow.

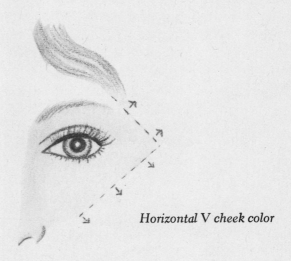

Horizontal V *cheek color*

"TOUCHING" WITH A PALETTE COLOR

Now is the time to "touch" your face in the earlier-mentioned spots, tapping and blending your palette color into the rest of your makeup.

PINK—MAGIC TRICK NUMBER THREE

Pink is a magic color for adding youth and life, for it brings a natural glow to any face. It must be added sparingly at the end of any makeup application and can be used in this manner effectively by all women regardless of coloring or makeup palette. The method of application is similar to the "touching" used in applying your palette color. Touch, tap and blend a soft (not pale) shade of pink into the following places: the temples, the center top of the forehead, just beyond the sides of the nose at the very beginning of the "apple" of your cheeks, just under your undereye concealer near the top of the "apple," the center of the chin and the earlobes. Youth is life, and life is pink.

POWDER

Always loose and always with a brush if you want to avoid an aged appearance. Never directly on any severely wrinkled area.

Powder is not a product with which you add color; if used at all, its purpose is merely to remove shine from the face. Select only a translucent powder (baby powder also works well) in either loose or pressed form. If you get loose powder, it can be helpful to put it in a salt shaker to facilitate getting the right amount into your palm. Put a small amount of powder into your hand and then, using a big, fluffy brush (tapping any excess powder out of the brush before you use it), fluff the powder, whisking the brush from side to side, down the center of your face with light strokes. If you prefer your powder in a pressed form, use the handle of the brush to draw a couple of circles lightly on top of the cake, loosening a small amount of the product. You now have, in effect, "loose" powder to apply as instructed above.

A LAST LOOK

When you have finished your entire makeup, examine it in a mirror by natural daylight. Stand next to a window and check to be sure you have achieved a balance of color and there are no obvious lines of demarcation. Your total makeup should create a total effect. The makeup itself should not draw attention away from *you*.

At this point in your development, because complete makeup application may be new to you, your time consumption may seem great. But once you get the knack of it, I promise you, the complete procedure will not take more than ten minutes.

Evening Makeup

Evening makeup is the same as daytime, except that everything should be stronger. Deeper shades can be used because the lighting will be more dramatic. The one caution here is not to overdo. Too much of anything creates a hard look, even on the very young.

If your eyelids are not wrinkled, evening is the time to use frosted eyeshadow.

Eyeliner can be deeper and directly match your eyeshadow—deep blues, greens, plums.

Black eyeliner pencil can be used to line the inner ledge of both the upper and lower eyelids *if* black eyeliner is used above and below the lashes as well *and* black mascara is used to finish the look.

Artificial eyelashes can be extremely effective at night.

Contouring can be more extreme at night because it isn't so apparent under artificial lights.

A light dusting of gold or silver powder with your big, fluffy brush can add a glow to the entire face (and/or hair) in the evening.

"Touching" the face with gold or silver in the same areas you touch with pink at the end of your makeup (right over the pink) can also add a lovely glow to the face. Lip gloss, tapped and blended well into the same spots on the face, can give the same effect.

Lip gloss mixed with a tiny bit of face glitter can become an interesting lipstick for evening. (A little goes a long way.)

Don't make the mistake of overdoing for evening. The goal is to intensify and dramatize, not to appear bright and shiny. Fad makeup styles for evening are almost always a mistake; one appears "costumey" or "freaky" rather than glamorous. It is one of the great sadnesses of our time that true glamour is missing from our culture. Glamour, especially heightened glamour created for evening activities of pleasure, is confident elegance. It is luxury in style, not in cost; it may glitter, but it is never gaudy; it marks the wonderful difference between day and evening, between production and consumption, between routine and romance. But evening makeup cannot do it alone, even if applied properly; it must be used to enhance evening clothing and an anticipitory attitude. Intensified and exciting makeup does not belong with the same clothes you would wear to the supermarket or an afternoon luncheon, no matter what the time of day. So save evening makeup for those special occasions that really call for it, or forego it altogether.

The No-Makeup Look

If you wish to create a no-makeup look, which I know many women prefer, you do *not* use less makeup. The trick here is to keep all of your color choices very close to your own natural coloring as well as very close to each other. Use all sparingly and blend well.

This means using a completely neutral foundation; soft (not light), subtle shades of cheek blusher in the brown family with just a touch of color; soft, subtle shades of lip color. It means ivory, beige and brown eyeshadows (no "color" colors), light brown, taupe or gray eyeliner and soft brown mascara.

Many women use this desire for the "natural" look to excuse themselves for simple laziness and neglect the makeup issue altogether. This is merely an excuse—it does not excuse. In order to achieve a natural look, a woman who wants to look younger must be more artful with makeup than ever. The only real color that should be used for a completely no-makeup look is cheek color, lip color and the pink (to add life and youth to any face) at the end of the makeup. All the rest must be achieved with beiges, ivories and browns.

One-Color Fast Faces

Once you become used to applying makeup, your everyday (full-face) makeup should take no longer than ten minutes—fifteen if you are very slow with your hands. Special-occasion and evening makeups, where your attention to detail is greater, may take a little longer.

However, there are times when there seemingly is no time for any makeup at all—a train to catch, getting a child to the school bus, etc. This is the time to utilize the one-color, fast-face technique. And it is the only time. This is not a substitute for a complete makeup, and it is not a lazy woman's way out of the makeup issue. If you wish to look younger, a complete makeup is the only way.

The one-color fast face uses, obviously enough, only one color. Keep on hand, for this purpose only, a dry blusher in your basic palette color but a few shades darker than you would use in your normal makeup routine—plum if your color is mauve, cinnamon if your color is bronze, deeper plum if that is already your color, etc. You will probably end up with a rather deep shade of one of the following: plum, rose, cinnamon, copper, brick or rust. Brushing this color on in different amounts will provide a healthy, alive, "attended to" look for your face without taking more than fifteen *seconds* of your time. Brush lightly onto cheeks (using the horizontal "V" placement) and heavily (but not *too* heavily) onto eyelids where your normal, medium eyeshadow would go. Next, wet your lips with your tongue and just touch the brush to them to leave a drop of color there and then finish off whatever is left on the brush by giving a fast swipe to your chin and the center of your neck.

If you have time to add undereye concealer and mascara, all the better.

Your Makeup Kit

In your purse, you should at all times keep a small makeup kit for touch-ups. Size, shape and color are optional, of course, but I find the small, transparent school bags with a zipper, which can be purchased in the dime store, the best. With these bags you can see at a glance the location of any item of makeup you need, and if by chance the bag becomes soiled, it can be washed easily with soap and water.

Inside the makeup kit, you will need a minimum of the following:

1 cream brown eyeshadow (to apply with fingers in order to refresh
    contouring or eyeshadow)
1 lipstick (to refresh lip and cheek color)
1 small blusher (optional)
1 undereye concealer
1 small pressed translucent powder (for *light* matting only)
1 pot or "crinkle stick" of eye cream (for keeping lines moist)
1 *small* (2" x 2") plastic bottle hand cream

The Always-Ready Bag

If you travel with any regularity at all, I also recommend keeping an "always-ready" bag in your travel drawer so that you need not address yourself to the subject of makeup and basic grooming products each time you travel, but simply drop the bag into your suitcase knowing that your every need has already been packed. This bag will have to be larger than your purse makeup kit, of course, and I think you will find it well worth the effort to have these products always ready. You will note that items already in your makeup kit are eliminated from this bag because you will presumably have your purse with you when you travel.

Inside the always-ready bag, you will need a minimum of the following:

1 foundation
1 blusher
1 eyeliner (if used)
1 mascara
1 eyebrow pencil (if used)
1 set eyeshadow makeup (either three basic, harmonizing colors or
    three shades of one basic color to emphasize your eyes, thereby
    going with all wardrobe changes)
1 pot or stick palette color

1 pot or stick pink-touching color

1 headband (for makeup application)

1 medium-sized, plastic bottle hand cream

1 plastic bottle skin freshener

Small plastic bag with a few cotton balls

1 jar each cleansing cream and moisturizing or protection cream
(kept in refrigerator between trips if made with natural vegetable oil)

1 small plastic jar fuller's earth (this can be made into a paste
with plain water for a quick beauty mask)

1 plastic bottle cologne

1 shower cap

1 plastic bottle shampoo

1 plastic bottle conditioner and/or rinse

1 razor

1 traveling manicure set (including two emery boards)

1 nail polish (for cover-ups)

1 small, traveling sewing kit (including safety pins)

1 small box pins, barrettes, etc., for hair

1 small hair (blow) dryer and/or rollers

A few packets Wash and Dry

1 small, wrapped (hotel-type) bar of soap

1 deodorant

6

THE MAGIC WARDROBE SCRAPBOOK

I call this eye-opener into the world of your wardrobe the "magic" scrapbook because after using it as a teaching aid in my beauty seminars, I have seen what magic it has performed for my students. Students of all ages, I might add. And students, too, who thought the idea was silly in the beginning, who declared loudly that they knew perfectly well their own clothing tastes . . . and who got surprised out of their ever-aging wardrobe ruts at the results.

The reason this scrapbook is such a successful learning tool, I believe, is that very few people ever fully conceptualize their wardrobe. Therefore, they wind up with an odd assortment of clothes, a collection lacking any coherent style or unity. Or, more commonly, they have nothing but repetitions of the same thing over and over again in their closets, and it would really make very little difference which selection they pulled from the rack.

By compiling a scrapbook—and updating it year after year—you learn what you really respond to, who you really are or strive to be and how to put it all together. Style is everything in dressing, but you need to be consciously aware of what you wish to stylize.

You also learn, after a longer period of time, how you change, how you (hopefully) grow and whom you are becoming. We change every year; the only question is whether or not we are aware of it.

116

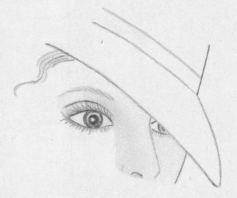

Compiling the Scrapbook

At this point, you should have accumulated a good number of clippings (from your magazines, remember?) in your large envelope. Your task now is threefold: You must *identify* the essence of the styles you have been drawn to through your clippings; then you must *evaluate* reality through examination of your own body and life-style; and, lastly, you must *act* to make your own personal statement through your clothing choices. Remember, you are never too old for this exercise. If, in fact, the key to a younger appearance is consciously creating your own individual look, it's even more important than ever that you devote some time and thought to this particular subject. A little hint: If you find yourself hesitating or resisting this idea, be *sure* you make yourself carry it out.

IDENTIFYING STYLE

Number One—Look through all your clippings, one at a time. If you come across anything that gives you a special sense of yourself (whether or not you think it has any connection to you or your own life), put a star in the corner of the page. In other words, if you see anything about which you could say, "If I were doing that, or wearing that, or could go there, I would really feel like *me*." Whatever stirs an excitement of that kind deserves a star.

Number Two—Label several sheets of plain paper with the following headings: 1. Dramatic, 2. Romantic, 3. Modern/Classic, 4. Casual, 5. Period/Costume, 6. Trendy.

Number Three—Lay your labeled sheets of paper out on the floor or a large table. Now place each separate clipping under the label that best describes it, or describes that which you like about it. If any particular clipping could go into more than one category, isolate the one attribute that is the *essence* of what you like and put it in that category only. In other words, if a gown is both "dramatic" and "romantic," decide whether it is primarily dramatic or romantic and put it in the dominant category.

You will probably end up with no more than two piles of clippings; many women end up with only one, which makes their task especially easy. If you have more than two piles, take the two largest piles and set them aside. Now go through your other lesser-filled categories and see if the clippings there can fit into one of your two major categories. You will most likely be able to reclassify the leftover clippings so that you end up with only two main categories. If you are unable to do so, decide how important the lesser-filled categories are to you. If they are less important than your two main categories, that will mean you won't eliminate that style altogether from your clothing choices, but you will save that alternate style for whimsical days when you feel like something different.

Group all clippings with stars on them together in each pile. Look them over separately and try to isolate the common denominator within them. Think of one word, if you can, that describes the thing they all have in common: "elegant," "fun," "quiet," "free," "romantic," "athletic," "sexy" are a few suggestions. Remember this one word when you select clothing to express your main category. Your choices should reflect the mood of that word as well.

(Using "Work Sheets" at the end of this book, keep notes as to your conclusions from the work you do in this chapter. Next year, when you repeat this exercise, you may find that the contrasts or similarities will provide you with more food for thought.)

If you find yourself with only one category, consider that *one* your basic style, the style that should thread consistently throughout all of your clothing choices in order to provide unity and identity (your identity) to *your* overall appearance. If you have two categories, decide which stylistic essence is most important to you (the difference in the sizes of the two piles may be an indication) and emphasize that style first. For example, my own personal style is "Romantic-Dramatic." I place the "Romantic" first because I have decided that romance is the primary essence of my style and that drama is strong enough to be included, but as a secondary consideration.

A note of warning: Before you run headlong into expressing your newly discovered style, give some thought to its veracity. Usually, when a woman comes to a stylistic conclusion through the use of this scrapbook method, she has a wonderful feeling of recognition. "Oh, yes, this really is me," or "I've always known it somewhere," or "I never realized it, but it's true," or "I never thought I could express that part of me here" or something of that nature.

If for some reason you experience a feeling of confusion or alienation from the style your scrapbook seems to push you toward, do not proceed any farther for the moment. Now you must give some strictly conscious thought as to what the essence of your style would be if you chose it conceptually. If it is different from that your scrapbook indicates, try to figure out why your conscious mind disagrees with your subconscious choices. Style is largely a subconsciously acquired phenomenon; it manifests itself in millions of little ways, from the way you pick up a phone to the way you make love—it's the way you come at the world in general and at yourself in particular. The expression of your own personal style should give you pleasure in all ways large and small, so don't impose upon yourself any stylistic choices that don't feel right. But if you sense a conflict here, don't ignore it either. Sit down and think about it. Psychology is outside the scope of this book, but the questions you ask yourself and the answers you find could be so useful in examining your own true style that the scrapbook will have more than accomplished its goal.

For the purposes of clothing, hair and makeup selections only—again, this is not a deep, psychological analysis—consider the following general hints to be applicable to your chosen style, and keep them in mind when evaluating your own fashion possibilities and needs.

Dramatic can get away with just about anything. It probably means you have a penchant for the unusual, the different. It means you like a variety of stimuli, even to the extent of some degree of incongruity. You can wear many things others cannot simply because of your daring and flair. You can wear inexpensive things well because your eye will lead you to extraordinary design. Be careful not to overdo; watch out for a tendency to come on too strong. This type is usually coupled with another category; let your second category lead you in all decisions of taste.

Romantic wants always to express an inner femininity. It could be the innocence of Victorian lace or the sexiness of a stripper's siren-satin; only you know how your own femininity feels to you. If you have placed yourself in this category, the important thing to remember is that your sense of romance is so strong you not only want to live it, but you want to exhibit it as well. You must, however, identify what form of romanticism expresses your own personal style of inner sexuality.

Modern/Classic usually expresses straightforward, but feminine, competence. If this is your category, elegance and quality are your guidelines. Clothes with easy wearability that do not detract from your abilities will express this stylistic essence. Be careful not to underdo. An understated look can be stunning, but you must be careful not to end up with a bored, "safe" look rather than one of classic quality. You may tend to require more expensive clothing because fine fabrics and cuts will be important to you. If cost is an issue, you will probably be happier with a small, quality wardrobe than with a larger one that does not really express your style.

Casual should lead you to an unstudied, country look. Comfort is probably most important to you, so look for freedom and mobility in your clothing choices. An unstudied look, however, takes plenty of study. Don't fall into the trap of laziness with this look and start to throw the style together instead of *put* it (consciously) together. A country or casual look can only be attractive if it bespeaks taste and quality. Well-cut designs with quality fabrics are a must in order to avoid a sloppy, careless appearance. And it *doesn't* mean jeans! (More on this later.)

Period/Costume is a form of romanticism, but rather than focusing on an inner romanticism (not that you don't have that as well), it centers itself more on a historical style. It could be anything from Victorianism to Orientalism to American Westernism, but whatever your interest, if it is strong enough to dominate your scrapbook, it should be expressed in your own stylistic choices as well. "Expressed" is the key word here, not "copied." The main pitfall to be avoided will be the tendency to look as if you were actually in costume. Remember that it is the style you are after, the feeling, not an actual return to some other period in time.

Trendy means you do not yet know yourself well enough to have acquired any particular style—even on the subconscious level utilized to compile your clippings. Assuming the age group that would be interested in a book with this title, it would be rare for anyone to select this category. However, if you have, do not despair. Go through your clippings again and *force* them into one or two of the other categories. This will at least give you a clue as to which direction you should head in clothing selections. If your clippings cannot even be squeezed into any of the other choices, you will have to compile another set of clippings, this time consciously directing yourself to select more personal images.

Glue your final group of clippings into a scrapbook, date the entry and redo this exercise each year (or keep it as an ongoing project—I do).

All types of categories should consider the next few points. Whatever basic stylistic category you have chosen (if you've come up with another one I have not listed and which better suits you, more power to you), it must now be personalized in order to express your unique individuality within the category. One woman's "Modern/Classic" will look entirely different from another woman's "Modern/Classic." Part of this goal will be accomplished by adapting your chosen style to your own body and life-style, discussion of which follows next. But part of the goal can also be accomplished by avoiding certain clothing choices altogether (or at least by exercising extreme caution when selecting them), which absolutely, and objectively, prevent a personal statement in appearance.

I must say that I am most sorry to have to bring certain of these particular clothing choices to your attention at all. I had hoped that at least the first two would all be out of fashion by the time of this writing, but since they are not, I am compelled to address them. No book, at this particular point in history, can hope to help any reader toward an individualized appearance as long as these "group" uniforms are popular.

Jeans—Here I am speaking primarily of blue jeans made of denim fabric. (A jean "cut" of different color and fabric is an entirely different matter, although any of this category, too, will always be, by the nature of its cut and stitching alone, suited for casual attire.) Contrary to popular belief, blue jeans do not "go" everywhere. Or at least they should not. Consider the place to which you are going. The ballet is a formal art. Jeans do not belong in the audience. Restaurants with tablecloths on their tables and which serve fine food have gone to some effort to prepare both food and ambience; you should go to some effort with your appearance in return. Unless your host or hostess specifies a "wear anything" evening, the same thought should go into your choice of dress as should go into their preparation for your entertainment. The point is that blue jeans are extremely casual, by nature of their cut, stitching and fabric. There is an issue of suitability here. If you insist on wearing blue jeans, consider whether they are really appropriate or not each time you wear them.

Further on this subject. Almost no one—of any age, but especially adults—looks good in blue jeans. Unless you are very tall and slim, they are usually not at all flattering. Start looking at most women wearing jeans from the back. That is probably what you look like, too. (This whole subject pertains to men as well.)

Lastly on this issue, there is nothing available in today's fashion world that proclaims total lack of individuality as completely as blue jeans. If you wish to look like *you*, whoever you are, you cannot do it by looking like everybody else from the waist down. If you think the name on your jeans makes any difference, read on, for you fall into the next category as well.

Designer-signature clothing—The inappropriate and constant wearing of blue jeans may proclaim either lack of individuality or laziness as stated above, but the insistence on designer signatures or initials on clothing signals something even less commendable: lack of confidence. If you need to advertise either the cost of a garment or the stamp of approval of another person (in this case the designer), you are automatically diverting attention away from yourself and onto the clothing itself. Clothing can be used very effectively to express your individuality; if you choose to emphasize someone else's personality with your choices, it is a clear indication that you, for whatever reason, choose not to "go it alone." Any woman who is sure of who she is and knows she is worth getting to know does not rely on status-symbol clothing to open doors for her.

Polyester fabrics—The only liability of wearing polyester (as far as trying to make a personal statement in your dress goes) is that much of it looks cheap and a good deal of clothing made with this fabric is poorly cut and finished. This is not an attempt to make you shy of polyester; its wrinkle-free aspects make it a wonder fabric indeed, and in combination with other fabrics it can be a real bonus. Just be careful in selecting it, looking always for quality and subtlety. There is nothing as unindividualized as jeans except all of the lime green, yellow and hot pink polyester skirt and pant suits walking down every main street in middle America. This particular look is aging as well because it has become connected with a matronly look that can make even the young look older.

Accessories—Slung over the polyester pant suits, you will usually see a vinyl handbag. Once again I caution you, this does not mean to stay away from vinyl altogether; it just means to be very careful when buying it. If you wish to achieve a distinctive appearance, you must stay away from the trap of buying, without thinking, what everybody else is buying. (Note the latest bore of carrying bags made of parachute nylon.) Let the style and shape of your accessories determine your choices, not their availability or price. It would be better to own one, lovely bag that you love than a dozen that do not express your stylistic category. The same goes for belts, scarves, jewelry, hats and gloves. Please don't misunderstand; I am not urging you to purchase only leather and real gold. Other fabrics and metals or plastics can be wonderful. I am, however, urging you to take great care and give conscious effort to the selection of accessories, for if *they* bespeak lack of personal taste, your appearance will suffer no matter what else you may be wearing.

One last word of warning to all types. The biggest backfire in "youthening" your appearance through clothing selections is to try to dress young. Nothing will make you look older. The young in *age* are, rightfully, experimenting before our very eyes. They are still identifying who they are and what they might like to become. Trends or fads are wonderful for them, no matter how crazy they may seem to be. Even the young look terrible, from the point of view of taste, a good deal of the time, but the blessing of each fad is that it soon passes. On an adult— precisely because trendy clothes and fads are identified with the young— the slavish following from one trend to another appears to be an attempt to *look* "young" rather than an attempt at experimenting. If you remember the ludicrous sight of all those fifty-year-old ladies in denim pant suits with sequin paintings on them several years back, you will know instantly what I mean. I repeat, the only way to look younger is to look like you. As you keep your scrapbook up, if you notice a change in the emphasis or the direction of your own personal style, *then* is the time to adjust your clothing selections. And you will do it, I guarantee you, because as you change and grow, your style will change right along with you. The only way you can ever look old or dated is if you don't keep up with yourself.

EVALUATING REALITY

Now to the task of evaluating the reality of your own body. Your chosen style must be expressed in the clothing you wear, true; but don't forget that it has to be worn on *your* body. Following are some general hints as to the types of designs that will look best on certain body shapes. They should be considered seriously when making actual selections. A slinky, Garbo-style gown may express your own romantic style, but will it look attractive on your five-foot-three, one-hundred-thirty-five-pound frame? Your style must be adapted to reality.

Measure your bust, your waist and your hips—bust across the tip of the nipples and around your back at the same level and hips seven inches below the waist. The ideally proportioned figure will show the bust and hips relatively the same, with the waist ten inches smaller. If you are top- or bottom-heavy, remember this when selecting clothes and balance the heavier section with fullness in the opposing section.

Tall and Slim Figures

1. Avoid severe, tailored lines in order to avoid a "spidery" effect.
2. Add curves to the body contour with soft, full fabrics.
3. Break the long line with a wide belt or contrasting color.
4. Create top interest with an overblouse or tunic.
5. Keep skirts circular or softly pleated to feminize look.
6. Wear hemlines slightly on the longer side.
7. Select fabrics with body and texture (such as mohair or tweeds).

Tall and Full Figures

1. Soft but tailored fashions will add fluidity to heaviness without adding fullness.
2. Avoid shiny fabrics and choose low-keyed colors to deemphasize size.
3. Vertical lines slim fullness.
4. Keep trim to a minimum to deemphasize heaviness.
5. Midwidth, self-fabric belts act as slimmers if the body is "full," not "fat."
6. Slightly flared skirts or straight but loosely fitted skirts soften without adding bulk.
7. Keep jackets two inches below the hipline to deemphasize hips but not draw attention to heavy derriere.
8. Medium, well-spaced patterns in darker, low-keyed colors can create movement to detract from fullness.

Short and Slim Figures

1. Rows of verticals with tucks or darts create both height and fullness.

2. Unbelted, Princess lines or Empire lines create length and curves of softness.

3. Side detail adds width without shortening line.

4. Short jackets add fullness.

5. Slightly flared skirts on the shorter side add softness.

6. Small patterned prints with same color trim add movement without overpowering.

7. Subtle colors increase curves.

Short and Full Figures

1. Vertical lines slim and lengthen lines.

2. Center closings accomplish the same.

3. Monotone ensembles deemphasize size while lengthening.

4. Basic, muted colors deemphasize size without shortening.

5. Slightly flared skirts worn a little on the long side slim without adding fullness.

6. Minimum of jewelry and accessories keeps appearance pared down.

7. Dull-surfaced, medium-weight, solid fabrics deemphasize extra weight.

Overweight Figures

1. One-color ensembles deemphasize size.

2. Clean, uncluttered looks do the same.

3. Longer hemlines act as slight slimmers.

4. Covering arms deemphasizes any flabbiness.

5. Simple capes, wide necklines and caftans deemphasize bulk and create interest in the face.

6. *Do not* wear clothes too tight or wear horizontal lines!

Tips for All Figure Types

1. Avoid clothing that is too tight—nothing makes angles, bumps or bulges more obvious.

2. Large legs can be camouflaged easily with pants or boots.

3. Create interest in your best assets by focusing attention there and detracting from less attractive points.

4. Do not wear street-length coats over evening gowns. If you do not have a special evening wrap, wear a simple shawl or cape. And do not carry a pocketbook with an evening dress. If you do not have an evening

bag, put your lipstick and comb in your gentleman's pocket, but a daytime bag looks absurd with an evening gown. (Don't laugh—I have personally spent evenings with wealthy and otherwise sophisticated women who have appeared in evening gowns with both pocketbook and raincoat.)

5. Be very careful purchasing shoes. If you are heavy, choose shoes with some "body" to them; otherwise you will look as if you are going to topple over in your high, spindly heels. If you are small, select unfussy, simply sleek styles; otherwise you will look rooted to the ground. Your height doesn't matter nearly as much as your overall body mass and structure. Also, note the way your legs look in any particular style; shoes should flatter the legs; for example, if you have short legs, ankle straps are not usually flattering. If comfort is most important to you, be extra careful to search out shoes that still exhibit style; nothing will age you sooner than wearing nurse-type shoes or flat heels just to be comfortable.

6. Select sleeves that cover flabby upper arms.

7. Exercise extreme caution in selecting necklines. A rounded scoop, in particular, can be aging, especially if it is elasticized. Any neckline that exposes any lined area of the chest must also provide some detail or unusual cut in order to detract from these physical age signs. And if you have wrinkles on your neck, be careful that the neckline does not draw attention to that area; if you have an extremely wrinkled neck area, turtleneck or cowlneck sweaters (provided your face is not heavy) and scarves around the neck can perform wonders in covering that area, thus hiding those signs of age.

8. Do not wear clearly out-of-date styles. Now, this bears a little elaboration. If you style your clothing choices to express your individuality, your chances of clothes going out-of-date before they wear out is minimal. However, it can happen, so watch for it. Coats in general, and furs in particular, can run the risk of becoming dated. This does not mean, per se, that you will look older, but it can mean that you give the impression of remaining in the past, which is a subtle sign of age. I hesitate to mention the subject at all for fear of being misunderstood to mean that you should follow fashion trends. I do not mean this. However, if a particular style, even though it may express you perfectly, is, in fact, also a *trend*, you must leave it when the trend is over—because the trend is outdated. If the clothing style itself has a short life (as for example, certain types of mink stoles or coat cuts or shoe styles), you must be extra careful in keeping it for yourself beyond

its own timelessness. Many styles, of course, never go out-of-date. These styles are the ones in which to invest your money.

9. Prescription glasses and sunglasses are also articles of clothing. They must be selected with enormous care. The pitfalls will be to look either trendy or out-of-date, either one of which will draw attention to your age. This is a legitimate problem because there are only so many styles available and they change all the time. But glasses (especially prescription eyeglasses that you wear a good deal of the time) are an unusual category in that they marry the aspects of both makeup and clothing. Since they become part of your face decor, they must be considered part of your makeup (your eye makeup should be much stronger if you wear glasses), but because they exhibit a particular style, they must also be considered an added touch of clothing.

Aside from expressing the style you have chosen for yourself, you should consider the following when selecting either prescription glasses or sunglasses:

LENSES

Even if you do not have to wear glasses to see images clearly, be sure the lenses of any type eyeglasses are of good quality. Cheap lenses (prescription or not), with any distortion, will cause your eyes to strain in order to see clearly. This strain will result in tired eyes, which will make anyone look older.

COLOR OF FRAME

Consider first the color tone of your own skin. If it is olive or sallow or very pale, you can add life to the entire face by selecting frames in *warm* colors—plums, ambers, rusts, etc. If your skin tone is anywhere in the ruddy category, *cool* colors such as greens, blues or grays will calm your own highly toned skin. Aging skins can benefit from warm but subtle and light colors, staying away from neutrals such as brown and gray. If you select a color that drains your own facial color, you will end up, once again, with a tired look that only adds years.

SHAPE OF FRAME

I cannot, here, describe in complete detail precisely what shape frame goes with which face because the individualities of every face shape are too diverse. However, there are a few general hints to be remembered. First, consider your own face structure; if your features are sharp and pronounced, they can be softened by fluidity in an eyeglass frame. The size and shape of your nose should be considered. Note the line of your natural eyebrows; your frames should follow that line—at the same level or perhaps just slightly above—to avoid what can look like wearing *two* sets of eyebrows, your own and the glass frame providing conflict of line.

SHAPE OF YOUR FACE

Round faces can benefit from square or straight-lined frames; square faces should be softened with rounded frames; a triangular face should take frames that deemphasize the widest section.

There has been very exciting progress made of late in the category of bifocals, always an obvious indicator that a woman has entered her later years. Newly perfected eyeglasses in this category, with "progressive addition" or "variable focus" lenses, connect the reading and the distance portions of the lens with an undiscernible band of gradually strengthened optical power; therefore, cosmetically speaking, with these new lenses it is virtually impossible to tell that you are the wearer of (horrors!) bifocals. It goes without saying that you should consult your doctor before embarking on any new prescription venture.

In another area, too, new designs make living with glasses easier. One of the questions repeatedly asked during the question-and-answer periods of my beauty lectures is how to apply makeup to the eyes when you can't see your eyes without glasses. This question always gets a laugh from the audience, but to an eyeglass wearer it's no laughing matter. Happily, there is at least one new product on the market to relieve this perplexing problem. Glasses are now available in which each lens folds separately down on the cheek, so that you can fold one lens down and apply makeup to the exposed eye while seeing clearly with the other eye through the other lens. Perfectly logical and perfectly wonderful for the women who have suffered up until now from misapplied makeup resulting not from lack of know-how, but simply from the fact they couldn't see to get the stuff on.

A note of warning concerning sunglasses: If you want to protect your eyes from glare and fatigue—not to mention the wrinkles—caused by squinting, choose dark lenses in the green or gray or perhaps brown category. "Fashion" glasses are fine to wear as color accent, but they do not protect your eyes.

Glasses—whether prescription or sunglasses—are important features of your overall appearance. Go at the subject with both eyes open.

10. Jewelry is a great attractor. Wear it, consciously, where you wish to draw attention . . . a stunning belt buckle on a trim waist, rings on beautiful hands, earrings to draw attention to the face, a droplet of a gem to focus on the breasts . . . but remember that the reverse is also true. If you wear jewelry indiscriminately, you will either divert the

viewer's attention entirely or attract the eyes to a feature you could do just as well not highlighting. And too much of anything is a bore. Be selective.

One other word of warning when wearing or purchasing jewelry. Be careful of getting fad jewelry (oh yes, it comes in gold and diamonds now) that will look out-of-date in a couple of years. Also, if everybody else is wearing chain necklaces, for example, and you *choose* to wear one as well, pay attention to the length of it in relation to the size of your face and the length of your neck. Many women (and *especially* men!) wear short, heavy chains around their necks that do nothing except make their faces look heavy and their heads chopped off from the rest of their body. Also, if you wear a short chain and you have wrinkles on your neck area, it will just draw attention to them.

11. When selecting stockings, panty hose or other, to wear with any particular outfit, be sure the color tone of the hose is in harmony with the color of your clothing—and do not wear daytime hose with evening clothes. Gray stockings, for example, will not look well with an all beige and brown outfit, unless you are accenting throughout with gray. Keep texture in mind as well. Nubby, textured hose do not go with soft jerseys and strappy sandals. You must have several different color tones available in your hosiery wardrobe, versatile enough to go properly with whatever you may be wearing on any particular day or evening; cost cannot be an issue today with all of the perfectly fine hosiery available to you from sources as near at hand and inexpensive as your local supermarket.

Instant Youth for All Figure Types

1. Wear support or control-top panty hose and nothing else underneath. For some reason many women do not realize that panty hose are designed to be worn without panties underneath them. They are meant to be worn for one day and then laundered just like all lingerie; that is why they all have a softer fabric in the crotch area. If you wear panties underneath, you ruin the very sleek line panty hose can afford you. And as instant "youtheners" they can work miracles. Especially under slacks or soft-fabric skirts, they become instant slimmers and firmer-uppers, helping to smooth out any bulges and giving the appearance of firm muscle tone at the same time. One note of warning: If you wear support panty hose with skirts and shoes rather than boots (so that your legs show), be certain your hose are sheer, sheer, sheer. Otherwise you will accidentally age yourself while using a youthening trick; opaque

stockings, unless specifically colored, have an "old lady" connotation, so make sure yours are silky and transparent.

2. Wear a bra. And wear one that *naturally* lifts your breasts into the youthful line they once had. This does not mean creating an artificial, padded look or an unnaturally pushed-up line, but just a simple lift that will, by lifting your breasts up from your chest, widen the area between them and your waist. This will make your waist appear smaller and your overall appearance trimmer and more youthful. If your breasts are naturally high or slope beautifully, the no-bra look may be perfectly fine for you; but if your breasts have begun to sag, a properly fitted bra (avoid the one-size-fits-all styles) can lift you into a proud, young position immediately.

3. Scarves can be utilized in a variety of ways to connote youth. Stylistically, they impart a carefree feeling—as if you are ready for a boat ride or to climb behind the wheel of a convertible—that presents a youthful attitude. They can be worn with great success around a neck that has begun to show its age. Around a waist just a bit too large to do justice to a belt (because the ends of the scarf flow downward, drawing extended attention away from the waist itself). Around hair (worn in a headband manner, which also pulls the face back, providing an instant face-lift; just make sure you leave the ends flowing over a shoulder to provide the spirit of youth as well). Around your entire head if your hair is not presentable (just be sure to add the interest of earrings and choose colors carefully so you don't end up looking like an old washerwoman). Or even tied carelessly around the strap of a handbag to add a dash of daring (as if you would be ready for the boat ride if one came along unexpectedly). One caution: Unless you have a *very* good eye and hand, it is best to avoid chiffon scarves. If the fabric is at all carelessly woven or flimsy in appearance, it will add years to you simply by looking old itself. Chiffon in any case works only as a long, flowing accessory that very few women can carry off anyway. Scarves of silk, fine cotton and good synthetics, however, have a marvelous ability to combine function with the stylistic spirit of youth.

4. Fluidity of fashion can serve the same purpose as a scarf, while adding a distinctive function of its own. Movement creates diversion. If your clothes have, among their other attributes, a quality of movement, via either the softness of fabric or direction in texture or pattern, a viewer's eye does not have the opportunity to rest for long on any one point of your figure. Now, you must be careful here. Subtlety is your watchword; otherwise you will keep your viewers' eyes so busy, they

won't have time to notice *you*. A "busy" print will backfire by distracting your viewer's attention, but fluidity of design or fabric can help keep another's eyes moving until they reach the most important resting place—your face.

5. Design cuts, patterns, focal points that have a quality of lifting the attention from either figure flaws or the lines of age can be extremely advantageous. As you will read in chapter 9 on hair, any cut that lifts the hair up and away toward the upper half of the face can aid in balancing the downward direction of age lines on the face. The same can be accomplished with clothing choices. With age, unless you have kept yourself physically fit, gravity begins to pull all the lines of your body down. This can, of course, be prevented or corrected with exercise. But until or unless that is forthcoming, any clothing designs that focus the attention upward, toward the upper half of the body and the face, can prove most successful in lifting the body into a youthful posture.

6. Wear pink. Or soft rose. *Not* a pink dress, or coat, or evening gown. But a pink scarf, a rose-pink blouse or sweater, a pink flower, rubies or other pink jewelry at the throat or as earrings. A touch of pink in your clothing can create instant youth in the same way—and for the same reasons—as touches of pink can bring instant youth to your face as a last drop of makeup. Obviously, I don't mean hot pink and I also don't mean lots of it, but a subtle touch of the soft glow of pink can bring life and youth to any style you may have chosen for your very own.

7. Make use of the "little black dress." This fashion selection used to carry the connotation of safety because it was worn when you didn't know quite *what* to wear. But not today; black is sexy, it is dramatic and it is, above all, slimming. Be sure to wear stronger makeup colors whenever you wear all black, make use of a pink or rose accent touch close to your face and don't forget to keep your shoes and hose in close color harmony.

8. Wear slimmer belts. Especially if your breasts have begun to droop at all (even though you wear a proper bra), the span between your waist and your breasts may seem to be shrinking. Poor posture can also contribute to this effect. Whatever the reason, a narrower belt—one or one and a half inches wide—will define the waist area and add slimness and length to the upper torso as well. If you wear an overblouse, try to use a slim belt or tie of the same fabric to define the waist without breaking the line.

9. Do not carry your handbag over one arm with the arm crooked at the elbow and crossed in front of you. You may have noticed that in

many "before" photos of make-over subjects the woman is standing with one knee slightly bent in the old 1940s Miss America stance and carrying her handbag in just this manner. This is an "old lady" look that can add years to anyone. If your bag has handles, grasp them in one hand and swing it naturally at your side as you walk. If you seem to need your hands free a great deal of the time, consider a shoulder bag instead.

10. Avoid all "little girl" decorations and mannerisms. Nothing points up a woman's mature years like wearing barrettes and ribbons in her hair or wearing "sweet" ruffles and rosebuds on her clothes. In the mannerism category, cuteness is usually off-putting, while confidence is enticing, and this includes pitch and timbre of voice. Many women *sound* like little girls (if anybody has ever asked you for your mommy when you answered the phone, this is a good clue you may fall into this habit category), which only emphasizes the distance between how they sound and how they look. Remember, little-girl tricks only work for little girls (unless you're looking for a daddy instead of a man, or a mommy instead of a friend).

Acting to Express Your Own Individual Style

Now it is time to put all that you have learned into action. It does absolutely no good if you have determined that you are Casual/Country on the inside unless you decide how to express that style with city clothes. Or vice versa.

The best way to begin to shape a style for yourself is to experiment. As suggested in your "shopping for clothes" activity, go to the best stores in your town. This way you will become acquainted with better designs and fabrics and cuts (not all expensive clothing is tasteful, heaven knows, but your chances are better for learning here than at your local discount center). Obviously, you do not have to *buy* here, and even if you can afford it, I do not suggest you buy new clothes just yet. Concentrate for the time being on restyling your own clothes, if that is possible, until you become more comfortable with this yet unfamiliar look and more facile at making new choices which express your chosen category.

You must learn, now, how to express your inner style on your outer body. Remembering the ten-inch contrast between bust and waist, and waist and hips, note the proportion and balancing effect different clothes afford you. Remembering those aspects of your body that you wish to emphasize or deemphasize, note which types of designs send attention to the focal point of your choice. Think how you can adapt a look to express your inner style if it seems difficult. For example, if you are tall and full, you will require a tailored, unfussy suit. But you can beautifully express your "romantic" style by adding a soft, flowing scarf to the neckline or carrying a long-haired fox muff. Remember, you do not have to be the walking embodiment of your style; but for your own pleasure in feeling like yourself (and for the hint you can give others trying to catch a glimpse of the inner you), you should try to adapt or add or revamp until your *overall* appearance expresses your chosen style. It is not as difficult as it sounds. Once you have consciously identified the style itself, the results can be achieved much more easily than you think.

Another way to help integrate what you have learned is to begin judging others. By looking at other women, see if you can identify their styles. Most of them probably won't have one—most women don't— but some will, consciously or not, and it can sharpen your eye to determine how they have achieved it. You must begin to train your eye. Note, on other women, what is helping and what is hindering their different figure types, etc. Go to the most expensive restaurants (for a drink only, if you wish) and observe how the women there have created their own styles. Money doesn't buy taste, certainly, but it sometimes buys these women the services of professionals who may have taste. Many wealthy women spend a fortune on hairstylists, clothes and personal grooming; it's possible for you to learn by noticing and identifying what they are doing right—or wrong.

When watching television, especially talk shows, observe the clothing and hair choices of women who seem to have a sense of style. Conversely, note obvious mistakes. You will find it shocking, if you consciously observe them, how many women who have the opportunity to be "in the know" don't know what to do with themselves.

Knowing what to do with yourself, however, does not mean doing it without consideration of your life-style. If you work long hours or spend much of your time chauffeuring children to and fro, you must remember, even though your style may be "romantic," that you need mobility and comfort as well. If you travel a good deal, your clothing choices should take into account fabrics that can save you time and trouble. A wise wardrobe not only expresses your exciting inner essence, it also expresses your ingenuity in making it realistically compatible with not only your body but your life.

When looking for compatibility, don't forget to consider color in your clothing selections as well. Bright, primary colors, for example, can run the risk of calling attention to themselves rather than to the person wearing them. They also focus attention on the torso, so if yours is a little heavy, it might be best to avoid them. Dark (and this doesn't mean only black), subtle colors diminish size (just as makeup does, remember?), and pale, light colors augment, so color can be an enormous aid to you in adapting your style to your given realities. As mentioned earlier, a drop of pink or rose will always achieve a youthful effect if worn close to the face. Solids, rather than prints, are safest for a few different reasons. First, the cost of the garment is harder to determine; cheap prints stand out like sore thumbs. Secondly, if there is a figure defect, solids can camouflage it through color alone, and you will make fewer mistakes in taste by selecting solids. Prints, no matter what the cost, are extremely difficult to choose. If you can do it competently, they can be helpful because they create movement, as mentioned earlier in this chapter; but if you err in any direction, the down-side is greater. For some reason, most prints look as if they would look much better hanging in the living room as draperies or in the kitchen as curtains. The major clothes categories for pitfalls are dresses, evening gowns and bathing suits—so many of them seem to have come from the upholstery department instead of ready-to-wear. The choices of prints in blouses is much better, but even there, caution must be exercised. I suppose the best hint here is to ask yourself if the garment would look well framing a window; if the answer is yes, pass it by.

On the Issue of Appropriateness

Once you have identified your personal style, you will naturally want to incorporate it into your entire wardrobe. Don't make the mistake of expressing yourself through your clothing on special occasions only. On the other hand, don't neglect to provide yourself with enough clothing categories, winding your individual style throughout, so that you can alter your basic look according to suitability.

Along with the loss of real glamour in today's world, which I touched on earlier, there seems to be a serious lack of appropriateness in dress as well. I mentioned this issue briefly in relation to blue jeans, but it is much more pervasive than that, and the subject deserves attention from anyone who wishes to dress well.

Americans, in particular, often seem to exhibit a total absence of appropriateness in their dress. Just walk into any airport; most of the travelers look as if they have arrived for a backyard barbecue. I have had guests who know that I prepare formal dinners with many elegant touches arrive in turtlenecks, pants and Western boots, looking for all the world as if they should be going to a rodeo. On the other hand, if you have been invited for an afternoon of swimming, boating and a cookout, it doesn't make much sense to wear three-inch heels with which to ruin the decking of a boat and twist an ankle. Your clothing for a weekend in the city should be different from that for a weekend in the country.

Aside from the poor taste and lack of thought displayed by inappropriate dressing behavior, if you do not vary your wardrobe according to the context of where you are going, with whom and why, you are missing out on a great deal of fun clothing-wise. It is boring to you and to those who have to look at you to *always* wear some form of a dress or pants or boots or whatever you're currently stuck on. In today's fashion world, more than at any time in the past, the variety of clothing choices is unlimited, offering an exciting array of not only styles but categories as well. Have style, yes, but to cling to only one or two categories is limiting and narrowing even if it perfectly expresses that style. Your clothing should not only express you, but it should also express your view of what you are doing and with whom and where you are doing it.

Think before you dress each day. Even if you work at the same job with the same people every day, you will perhaps be doing something different for lunch or after work that could influence your clothing choice on any particular day (this does *not* mean to wear evening-type clothing to work). If you're going to someone's home for a luncheon that includes a tennis game before lunch, you should dress differently than if there are plans for a card game afterward. If you look the same on Saturday morning as you do on Saturday evening, you are indeed cheating yourself—and others. Your attire should be appropriate to the occasion as well as to yourself.

There is one area, however, where (almost) anything goes. And that is in your own home, when you are the hostess. Even if it's a backyard barbecue, *you* can wear a strapless dress to your ankles and go barefoot. If it's brunch, you and you alone can wear an antique satin kimono. When it's your party, you are the star, and you should dress like one. This is the time to pull out all the stops—you can virtually do no wrong (except by wearing blue jeans to your own eight-course French dinner). At-home dressing can be fascinating, fantastic or fantasy. You can have a ball.

Even if there are no guests, you might consider dressing differently in the evening than you have all day long. Changing clothes, getting comfortable and pretty in some new way is a wonderful way to treat yourself to a change of attitude as well as attire and create a lovely feeling of anticipation even if the evening ahead promises nothing more exotic than a good book by the fire.

There are so many wonderful ways to add variety and grace not only to your appearance but also to your life-style through the simple method of clothing choices that I cannot imagine the boredom of wearing the same old look everywhere, every day. If you do, chances are you're not the only person you are boring.

Most women should have at least one choice in the following categories as a minimal wardrobe:

Pants—dress and casual
Shirts—solid and printed
Blouses—at least one silk- or satin-type fabric
Sweaters—dress and casual sweaters for indoors, plus an over-sweater
    for out-of-doors, plus one to wear casually as a light wrap
Skirts—dress and casual
Blazers—at least one to wear as a man wears a sportscoat
Dresses—dress and casual
Coats—everyday spring and winter, special occasion, raincoat, eve-
    ning wrap
Gowns—at least one "drop dead" gown (even if you wear it no-
    where but your own dinner table with a suitable guest)
Shoes—walking, dress, casual, evening, plus good boots and rain
    boots
Belts—dress and casual
Bags—day and evening
Gloves, Scarves—at least three of each
Robes—morning and evening with appropriate slippers
Nightgowns—at least one "drop dead" gown (even if you never
    wear it at all)

If, after looking over this very small list, you see that you have six pairs of pants and no skirts, four skirts but only one sweater and not a thing to wear on a dressy evening, you will see the gaps in your wardrobe. If you say, "But I never need anything dressy for evening," then there is more missing from your life than an item of clothing.

If various clothes categories are not present in your wardrobe, you will hardly be stimulated to vary your appearance by mixing, matching and trying new combinations. Be assured, if you stick to the same old thing in your dress, you will always look that way to others—the same old thing. If you want to look younger, even though you revamp your makeup and hairstyle, your wardrobe must express you first, yes . . . but it must also exhibit some energy and imagination. Be creative, give a boost to your life through your wardrobe, have fun.

On the Issue of Money or How to Dress Rich Even if You're Not

The single biggest mistake women with limited funds make in shopping for clothes is to go shopping where they can realistically buy. You should *buy* your clothes there, but you should not *shop* for them there.

I have asked you to read this chapter before you go out "shopping" tomorrow. This "shop" may be the first of its kind for you, and that is one of the reasons I am giving it to you as one of your ten-day program activities. If you do it only this one time, it will truly help you determine and become familiar with your newly chosen, personal style, or the one you will now be trying to acquire. But it is my hope that, unless you have an unlimited wardrobe budget, this method of shopping will become a useful tool in future clothing selections as well.

This mistake of shopping for only what you can afford is common with both men and women; and it cuts across all interests, all styles and all pocketbooks. If you train your sights on only that which you can realistically purchase, you automatically lower your sights stylistically. Find out first what you like. *Then* adapt and accommodate or alter according to your budget.

By shopping at the best stores you will begin to be able to judge fabric, design cuts, colors and style much better than if you confine your tastes by automatically heading where your purchasing power lies. Go to specialty shops, exclusive boutiques, posh little corners in ritzy department stores. Be sure not to become a slave to these choices either, of course; your motive is to learn to distinguish between originality and kitsch, classic styles and trends, good and poor fabrics and workmanship. Be advised that you can find junk everywhere, in fine stores as well as less expensive ones; no one has to be told that money can't buy class.

However, the quality will undoubtedly be higher at the fine store because the clients who buy there can, at those prices, demand (and get) more. They're paying for it. But you can benefit immensely from the selections offered there from a training point of view.

Sometimes you can even buy at these expensive shops. You'll find, if you frequent them every so often, that you can purchase a stunning item on sale (which would never even be available to you in a "normal" store) for no more money than you would ordinarily spend on a comparable—and less smashing—garment elsewhere. But, even if you don't ever buy a thing, keep going for the single purpose of advancing your taste.

If you sew, you really have an incredible advantage. You can go home and copy the garment for a tenth of its purchase price. Sewing, of course, is the best way to save money on a wardrobe because, since you are paying out of pocket only for the fabric, you can afford to select the finest fabrics available and also create whatever style you wish. However, even if you don't have that time or talent, a stylish, expensive-looking wardrobe can be yours inexpensively—if you know what you are doing. Shopping at fine stores is the first step.

You must know next how to select wisely at the stores in which you can afford to buy. Simple designs and cuts are a good guideline—your shopping sojourns will train your eye in this matter—as are solid, subtle colors and straightforward lines. If you purchase a simple wool skirt and your hands have learned from your shopping trips how to determine a quality "feel" in a fabric, it will be impossible for anyone else ever to guess the cost of your skirt. *This* is confidence in dressing. The cost of your clothes should not scream at a viewer, no matter where along the economic spectrum they were purchased. It is your style, your individuality that should be expressed, not that of the store where the purchase was made.

The wisest way to allocate money in wardrobe purchases is to save on simple, not-possible-to-classify clothes like the above-mentioned skirt. Inexpensive blouses are to be had by the dozens, as are inexpensive pants and shoes—*if* you have learned what you're doing. Distinguish these items with accessories, where it pays to invest more money because they will last longer—handbags, jewelry, etc. If you wear a simple little ten-dollar jersey dress (oh, yes—available, on sale, even today—*if* you have learned what you are doing), it will serve the same purpose of becoming a backdrop for a seriously purchased silver belt as a simple little one-hundred-dollar jersey dress. If you're going to spend money, make it count. If you have very little to spend on any item, let your educated eye and hands find impossible-to-categorize styles that bespeak simplicity and quality of design. You can shop in a five-and-ten and come out looking like Fifth Avenue—*if* you acquired your training on Fifth Avenue.

Experiment, experiment, experiment. You may make a few mistakes while you are learning, but your efforts will pay off; and it's still better to make mistakes while trying to look like *somebody*—yourself—than, like most women, looking like nobody at all, or *everybody* as the case may be. This last, I repeat, is the major reason other people's attention becomes focused on a person's age. If you make no personal statement with which to attract another's attention, that attention will naturally settle on the most obvious point—frequently, age. If, on the other hand, you create an external style to focus people's attention on your individuality, they will be far less concerned with irrelevant subjects such as what year you were born. Another point: Young people (young in age) spend a great deal of effort on their outward appearance. Even in this jeans age, they spend much time on hair and makeup. Lack of effort by an adult only indicates that she's grown too tired (old) to care.

You must care. But you must also care enough about yourself to express the real you.

7

SIGNATURE HAIR
(YOUR SIGNATURE)

Have you ever noticed how many women wear the hair "signature" of someone else? A famous hairstylist's latest creation, or a favorite public figure's latest style, or whatever is latest on the block—whether or not it suits the woman's own particular features or personality or life-style? Look around. Look in the mirror.

Of all adornments in the world, a person's hairstyle is probably the most important. It is one of the few natural adornments that you can easily and substantially alter and which you wear all of the time, with and without clothes, during all seasons and all weather. Why not make it yours?

The Anatomy of Hair

It will help you in making decisions about your own hair if you first understand the nature of *all* hair. It can hardly be cared for successfully if it is not understood.

There are some interesting myths about hair that are quite commonly accepted, so perhaps we should begin by correcting some of the more glaring ones. To begin with, there is a prevalent misconception that each individual hair is made up of a series of tubes, one nesting snugly inside the other. This is not the case.

The anatomy of hair is one not of tubes but of layers. The outer layer is clear and scaly; it is called the *cuticle*. The next layer, and actually the main bulk of the hair, is the *cortex* and is made up of fairly tough fibers bound together lengthwise.

The core of the hair shaft is the *medulla*, which may or may not be present. If it is, it can be made up of two or three or even four layers itself. The medulla does not concern us for the purposes of hair care, but I mention it simply because it must be included in any complete description of the hair.

On the outside of these three main layers (assuming the medulla is present) and forming a protective cloak at the surface of the entire hair shaft is the *epicuticle*. This is, technically, the outermost layer of the *cuticle* and is made up of flat, interlocking cells. It is the epicuticle that is of greatest concern to anyone addressing the subject of hair care. The epicuticle is cemented onto the main body of the hair shaft by a thin layer of protein. It is this protective layer of the hair that becomes damaged quite easily. And it is this layer that protein conditioners can sometimes repair by more or less "re-cementing" the coating of protein.

Another myth that must be banished here is the fallacy that the growing power of each hair is diminished if it has split ends. It is still the custom in Europe and used to be popular here to singe split ends with heat in order to "close" the "tube" and seal off the ends to promote growth.

What is done to the visible part of your hair certainly affects the condition and appearance of it, but there is no evidence to indicate that it actually affects growth. (Since singeing does eliminate split ends, the hair doesn't need to be cut so often, thus making it seem to grow longer; but the growing power of each hair is tucked firmly *below* the skin's surface.)

Each hair has a root that lies beneath the scalp, and that root contains a hair bulb; it is that hair bulb from which the hair grows. The hair, like the skin, lives out an ever-renewing cycle of growing the new and shedding the old. The new, and still-actively growing hair will lengthen somewhere between one-half and one inch per month. Once the hair itself is old, no matter how short you cut it or how often you singe it, its growing power will terminate, the root will die and the hair will be sloughed off. As each hair dies in a healthy head of hair, a new one replaces it.

Your hair has more growth energy in warm weather than in cold, which is the reason tinted hair needs more touch-ups in summer than in winter even if it has been protected from the bleaching rays of the sun.

Brushing the hair (unless you have an oily scalp) is a fine method to keep the mass of your hair free of old hairs, preventing them from falling onto your clothing and creating unsightliness.

A word should be said here about combing the hair. While brushing gently removes unwanted hairs, combing can pull out or break off healthy hair, so care should be exercised. Select a wide-toothed comb with oval spaces between the teeth. The points of the teeth should be rounded in order to avoid scratching the scalp. When you're combing wet hair, extra caution is necessary. Wet hair loses some of its elasticity and can be stretched (the curling process) and broken more easily.

Finely textured hair is more delicate than coarsely textured hair. The pigment, or natural color, of the hair is contained in the cortex layer. It is this natural color that determines the texture of your hair. Natural blondes—very little color—usually have fine texture. On the other end of the spectrum are redheads, with a coarse texture and lots of body, meaning a heavy cortex layer. Brunettes, depending on the depth of shade, fall somewhere in between.

Texture, by the way, is an important consideration in determining how much trauma your hair can withstand in any tinting process. One-process tinting is easier on hair in general than double-process tinting for the following reasons: The cuticle must first be softened and opened in order for the chemicals to penetrate the cortex and deposit new color. With a single-process, the lightening and coloring processes take place almost at the same time. The lightening action works first to open the cuticle and then find its way to the natural pigment in order to lighten it. As soon as the natural pigment has been lightened just enough to receive the new color, the coloring action takes over until the hair becomes the desired shade.

A double- or two-process hair coloring is used only when you want a dramatic change in color. The lightener is applied first to strip the hair of its natural color. Because it has a great deal of lightening to accomplish, it takes a while (usually around an hour) for the bleach to penetrate the cuticle scale and lighten the natural pigment. In some cases, it takes two applications of bleach to get the natural color out. After this is accomplished—causing great trauma to the condition of the hair—the new color is applied as a separate application. Chemicals are thus in contact with your scalp at least three times as long as with a one-process application.

Most hair-tinting processes today do a remarkable job at creating whatever color your heart desires with the least amount of trauma. However, I recommend a one-process color for two reasons. As described above, it is much easier on the condition of your hair. In addition, most hair colors that require a two-process application are terribly aging to the wearer. Artificial colors and pastel, cotton-candy-type unnatural shades add years to almost any face. It is true that lighter shades are more attractive on an aging face, but unnatural colors and shades have just the opposite effect.

While we are on the subject of color, there are two issues that must be treated, since the thrust of our efforts is to add youth to your appearance. The first is gray hair. In my opinion, if you have gray hair now, I can virtually guarantee a loss of several years immediately if you will only eliminate the gray. Gray hair is aging. To anyone. I cannot imagine how the myth ever gained a moment's notice; you know, the one that says *certain* shades of gray, or silver or white, are attractive. Well, they may be attractive to some—that is a subjective judgment—but they are aging to all. Men included. Perhaps the male side of this myth harks back to a time when women wanted a "mature" man, which usually meant money and security (a little dignity around the temples). But if you look honestly, the most obvious reaction to men or women with gray or white hair is that they are "older." Even if they aren't. Many men, especially, in their very attractive forties, age themselves terribly by leaving their naturally gray or white hair uncolored; they end up looking older than they actually are!

The amount or the placement of gray or white or silver (I will use them all interchangeably because they all result in the same effect) is really irrelevant. Some people, it is true, get gray hair very early in life, but usually gray hairs do not start popping up until one is past the half-way mark, so it is only normal for others to assume that you are older. Heaven knows, in past generations, before the Industrial Revolution, there was no choice but to go gray if Mother Nature and your heredity so dictated. But in today's wonderful world, there is no need. You can be any color—including your natural one—you desire. Hair color is now an act of will, not an act of nature. And this fact can be very helpful to anyone wanting to lose years. Be sure to select soft, subtle colors, as bright or dark colors, because of their harshness, are aging.

The second issue I want to battle is directly related. Since hair color can now be an act of will, it escapes me why so many women *create* gray hair for themselves by frosting their hair when even Nature hasn't wielded her streaks of age! The original purpose of frosting was to lighten the feeling of the natural color, thereby adding youth to a face without all of the fuss and trouble and money of actually tinting the hair.

Now, it is true that as a person's face ages, it often loses much of the color and life of youth. Therefore, a lighter feeling to the frame of the face, the hair, would have just that youthening effect. In fact, I absolutely recommend that as a woman ages a bit—perhaps in the fifties range—she lighten whatever color she may have had up until that time, whether her own or tinted, by one or two shades. It will buoy the facial complexion by lifting the color-life of the hair and act to erase years. But notice that I say to lighten the entire shade. Young hair has hundreds of varying colors in it to sum up in the one final color of hair that is predominant, meaning you can say, "She has red hair." But none of those colors is gray. Unfortunately, whatever the purpose of frosting may be, the result is usually some form or shade of age-streaked "graying" hair, which is just across-the-board disastrous to anyone's good looks, let alone her desire for a youthful appearance. It's like going gray on purpose when you shouldn't permit yourself to stay gray even if it happens naturally.

As far as the money is concerned, that is no reason to do a halfway job on yourself. If you are in fact going gray naturally, then the tinting process is actually easier. The presence of gray hair is nothing more than a manifestation of the absence of pigmentation from the cortex layer of the hair. That means that there is no longer any natural color present at all. Therefore, in order to tint such hair, no lightening process is necessary, simply the coloring process. This is why gray hair can be colored with very little trauma to the condition of the hair; and this is why, too, coloring shampoos or even temporary rinses can be so effective with hair that contains a fair amount of natural gray.

But halfway efforts in order to save the money of full tinting, because you don't have to do it so often, are no bargain if all you end up with is either the artificiality or the aging aspects of frosted hair. Unless you have a great deal of gold in your natural color—in which case, clever frosting can result in a natural sunkissed appearance—the whole phenomenon of frosting will usually backfire in every way. If you want the youthful benefits of a lighter frame around your face without the fuss or cost of regular tinting, I would suggest you go only one or two small and soft shades lighter than your natural color (covering all natural gray, of course), which will satisfy your desires to some realistic degree without requiring touch-ups on a frequent basis. However, ideally, I would always recommend coloring your hair exactly the shade you think is best for your own skin coloring and your own individual personality style and foregoing all shortcuts. If you can't do it for yourself, perhaps you and a friend could perform the service for each other (it's very simple), or you could simply exert the time and effort required, giving up something else financially to be able to afford professional care. But hair color and style are so important to anyone's looks, let alone someone who is trying to emphasize youth, that I think they deserve top priority on every modern woman's list.

Lastly, to conclude discussion of the physical aspects of your hair—keep it clean. As with the skin, cleansing is the single most important issue for the health and beauty of hair, whether virgin or violated, youthful or gray. Shampoo, preferably with soft water, as often as you feel it is necessary. If you have long hair or a light color or an oily scalp, you'll require frequent shampooing. It is another myth that daily washing affects the hair adversely or causes it to fall out.

Always end your shampoo with an apple cider vinegar rinse—½ cup vinegar and enough cool water to make a quart of rinse. Even if you use a conditioning treatment or a cream rinse, pour this apple cider rinse through afterward. It will restore the proper pH factor (between 4.4 and 5.5 for the hair) and at the same time separate the hairs so that each one can reflect the light and give your whole head a radiant luster.

Idiosyncracies of Your Hair

Every woman I have ever met is aware of the individual characteristics of her own hair. Most of us are dissatisfied with what we have—if it's straight, we wish it were wavy and vice versa; if it's fine, we wish it were thick, etc. However, these aspects of our hair are facts of reality. We can change color and length and style, but the actual physical characteristics of our hair we must learn to accept to some extent. If you have baby-fine hair, you may as well save yourself time, money and grief; even with a body-wave, you will never be able to wear a style that requires strength and a coarse texture. However, any style you prefer can be adapted to the individualities of your own hair. If for some reason you have not yet identified the following characteristics of *your* hair, do so now. You cannot successfully select a style that will work for you unless you take this knowledge into consideration.

Texture. As mentioned earlier, the natural color of your hair will give you a clue. There are exceptions to this rule, but usually the less color pigment, the less body your hair will have. Fine-textured hair may take a curl easily, but it will soon lose it and fall straight again. If your hair is dark and thin, you will also tend to have a sparse amount of hair. Examine your hair and decide if it is *fine, medium* or *coarse.* When selecting a style, remember that if you have fine hair, for example, you will never be able to achieve a full, heavy look to your hair. Discuss the limitations of your own texture with your hairdresser before you settle upon a final style.

Elasticity or Strength. If your own hair is not basically strong, you will have to remember to go gently with blow dryers, curling, straightening and bleaching. This can affect your decision when choosing a style. In order to determine this elasticity, pull out a single hair from your head. Using the index finger and the thumb of both hands, grasp each end of the hair and pull. If it snaps immediately, your hair will damage easily. If you can pull and pull and the hair seems to stretch for a long time before breaking, you could select a style that requires much harsher treatment to maintain.

Natural Curl. This is probably the most important attribute of your hair that will affect style choices. If your hair is completely straight, of course, you can always have a permanent—but probably not if you have fine hair that damages easily. (You begin to see how you must consider your hair before you can decide upon a style.) Wavy or curly hair can of course be straightened—but probably not if you tint your hair, which already subjects it to chemical trauma. Put your natural hair condition into one of the following categories: straight, slight bend, wavy, slightly curly, very curly, kinky. Discuss this aspect of your hair with your hairdresser before going ahead with one particular style. If you try for a style that goes against the nature of your hair, you may find that you have achieved only a headache instead of a hairstyle.

Selecting a "Signature" Hairstyle

In order to give a personal signature to your own hairstyle, you must, number one, be willing (or brave enough) to forget what "everyone else" is wearing or what you have always worn. And I encourage you to do so. If you look around at your acquaintances, I don't care what their financial or social status, you will be able, almost to the year, to determine when they last addressed themselves to the hairstyle subject. One of the fastest ways to date yourself is to adopt the latest hair fashion and then go on wearing it for years. There are women around today still wearing the teased, beige styles of the fifties. Others are still walking around with the shag look. The natural Afro still pops up in the grocery store, and I think every other housewife in Middle America is still wearing that short cut with bangs blowing up and away (which was great on the figure skater for whom it was designed, but is it for you?).

If most women have not rooted themselves in one outdated hairstyle, they have moved through the fashions adopting *each* new one, as it came along, regardless of its suitability to their own features or life-style. Your hairstyle is important. It deserves serious consideration and thought.

Consideration number one—What is your basic *figure* type? Short, tall, medium? Thin, average, heavy? Big- or small-boned? If you are short and thin and small-boned and try to wear a hairstyle that is big and "blowy" (unless you are a very dramatic type), you will appear to be "walking hair"; it will so overpower your basic stature that it will detract from *you*. If you are tall with a fuller figure, you can carry the larger waves and freer movement of a big style. If you are very tall and thin and select a short, straight "boy" cut, you may well end up looking like a preppy male youth approaching puberty.

Think about your basic body structure before deciding upon a hairstyle. What is your basic silhouette? If you have a photo of yourself standing in a bathing suit, cut your figure out of the photo. Next, trace the outline on a blank sheet of paper and then fill in the figure with a black, felt pen. Note your figure proportions. Make several of these silhouettes and play around with basic hair shapes by drawing in several different types of basic hair lengths and widths. Which ones complement your basic, overall stature? This doesn't mean that you have to duplicate the shape of the drawing on your head, but it will help to give you direction.

Whatever you do, be sure to consider your body shape *as it is now*. Even if you have maintained your weight and muscle tone, your body has undoubtedly changed proportionately in some way over the past years. Don't *remember* the way your body looks; look at it now. It may help to view your body as if it were that of a stranger in order to gain the objectivity you need.

Consideration number two—What is your basic face shape? Now don't take this literally; no one has an exactly square face, but once again, it will help to give you direction. The basic face shapes are as follows: round, square, oblong, triangle, heart (or inverted triangle) and diamond. Certain principles of hairstyling can be considered to generally enhance any particular face shape. Following is a list of those general principles. These are only guidelines and should not be followed slavishly any more than any latest fad should be followed slavishly. The whole idea behind achieving signature hair is to individualize any style considerations to yourself.

Round—Asymmetry can be helpful in order to throw emphasis to one side of the face or the other; consider a high, side part or bangs to cut off part of the forehead or long and straight at the sides to cut off the roundness. The principle here is to avoid adding width and to try to create angles in the face shape.

Square—This shape needs softness to feminize angles; do not add more width at the jawline; a high side part is possible, or some form of soft bang to cut off the squareness of the forehead. The principle here is to soften the natural angles of the face shape.

Oblong—Do not necessarily try to shorten the face, but be sure not to lengthen it further; side interest can draw attention away from the length of the face; a low side part is a possibility; greater width at the top of the head can act to slim the jawline. The principle here is to create horizontal or side interest.

Triangular—Add greater width at the top of the head to balance the wide jawline; bangs can camouflage the narrow forehead line. The principle here is to soften and balance in order to counteract the wide angle of the chin line.

Heart-shaped (inverted triangle)—Keep hair close to the head at its widest point; fullness below the ears can counteract the wide forehead; a center part that is slightly *off*-center can be particularly helpful especially with short wisps of hair left to softly cover the wide area of the forehead. The principle here is to draw attention to and soften the lower half of the face *or* narrow the widest section.

Diamond-shaped—Keep hair close to the head at the widest point; at the forehead cover only enough to camouflage the lack of width; and off-center part can be helpful, as can fullness below the ears. The principle here is to camouflage the angles.

As with your body, examine your face shape as it is *now*. As the years pass, facial contours change along with body contours. For example, did you know that the nose and ears continue to grow after the rest of the facial structure terminates its growth? Even if only a minute amount, this factor alone can alter your basic face shape. Weight and age will also have some effect. So, as with your body, be sure not to *remember* your face shape. Look at it as it is *now*.

General tips:

1. A long neck can carry longer hair; a shorter neck needs a modified length to bare what neck you do have and make it appear longer.

2. You can balance a nonstraight nose by positioning your part on the opposite side of the bend (gives the illusion of "bending it back").

3. Off-the-forehead hair lends focus more openly to the entire face.

4. Bangs can focus interest on the eyes and cover a lined forehead (as can tiny wisps).

5. Simple hairstyles divert attention away from the hair and onto the deeper personality of the wearer; fussy styles draw attention to themselves.

6. Any cut that emphasizes an upward direction can offer a lift to the face, thereby giving a youthful effect.

7. Soft, natural styles, without a "set" look are more youthful in appearance.

8. Unless your features are perfect and your face unlined, any severe style pulled completely back from the face will add years.

Your Hairstyle and Your Life-style

Your life-style may be the single most important consideration you will employ to reach your final decision in choice of hairstyle. If you are tending toward a complicated, wavy, must-be-set style, and you swim or play tennis three times a week, you may want to reconsider. It is usually better to adapt a style (or even select a second choice) to your particular context than to try to do the reverse. For example, if you have a demanding career, you may not have time to wash and blow-dry every morning. On the other hand, if you have plenty of time and entertain a great deal, you may do very well with a more complicated style. Think about this issue and be honest as to how much time and care you are willing to devote to your hair. It will help you determine your style, and will help your hairdresser adapt your chosen style to your life.

The Advantages of Wigs

As outlined in Day Five of your program, I recommend that after you have considered all of the previous suggestions in this chapter, you actually try a variety of styles. The very best way to do this is to experiment with wigs.

Be sure that you are dressed well and have applied a complete makeup before you go "shopping" (not for wigs, but for styles), so that you will look essentially the way you would with any of the styles or colors adapted to your own hair. Don't forget, too, that if you seem to find a basically interesting style, you can comb or brush the wig into slightly different styles in order to pursue a particular possibility. You are not endeavoring here to find the one wig that will look exactly like the one best hairstyle for you; rather, you are gathering still more information to help you determine which direction you will take in deciding your own, personal style.

The Last Step—Your Hairdresser

The reason that I recommend you go to a *new* hairdresser is because, if you wish to individualize and personalize your own hairstyle, it is better to see someone who does not know you already. Your regular hairdresser, if you have one, undoubtedly has made certain judgments about you that could influence his or her objectivity in helping you into a new style.

Once you are at the shop, sit down and discuss all that you have learned about your choice of a style and about your life-style. If your hairdresser will not discuss these matters with you—leave. I do not mean that you should expect a hairdresser to sit for an hour and listen to your life's history; but the motive behind all of the think-time you have already invested in this subject is to emerge with a hairstyle that is best for you and *right* for you. If your hairdresser will not take the time to assist you with his own expertise toward this end, you don't need him. If you find that you cannot communicate with your hairdresser, then you will most probably not receive a style and cut from him that will make you happy anyway. Remember, too, that many hairdressers are capable of performing only certain, locked-in sets. If you want something and he tries to steer you away from it, it *could* be because he doesn't know how to do it.

A hairdresser's function for you is to help you adapt the style you think you would like to wear to your own hair. If he thinks of some legitimately negative reason why this style wouldn't be best for you, that, of course, would be extremely helpful, because it would prevent you from making a mistake; or he may be able to adjust the style to make it better for you. One other tip: If your new style requires any expertise in setting or blowing out, have your hairdresser show you how to do it before you leave. A blow-dryer in the hands of a professional is quite different from you, alone, wrestling with the machine at home.

One last reminder: If your hair is not quite what you expected or wanted after the first cutting, do not despair. Even if your hairdresser is perfectly cooperative, he is not superhuman. If the basic style is what you both were after, he can refine or correct it during future cuttings. And if you have made a serious mistake in your choice, you can redo it at some later date (it is not the end of the world), and at least you will still have accomplished an important goal; you will have lifted yourself out of the mass of lookalikes and begun down a road that will have delightful rewards at the end. You will have begun to look and feel like yourself, and your hair will at last carry your own signature.

8

A SPORTING CHANCE

First of all, don't say, "I'm not athletic," and skip this chapter. I'll deal with you at the end of it. So read on. . . .

Some of my more astute readers will have noticed that the chapter on Wake-up Warm-ups is very short. They will also have noticed that I do not admonish any woman to perform extensive exercise routines every day. There are two major reasons for my particular approach to the subject of exercise. One is that anyone truly interested in a complete program for a regular exercise regime should purchase a book dealing strictly with that subject alone. Only such a book, devoting its entire attention to the full spectrum of physical exercises per se, could delve into the depth of their particular benefits and offer instructions in the detailed way necessary to make any treatment of the subject really worthwhile. Therefore, a complete analysis on my part would be outside the scope of this book.

But there is a larger reason, and that is as follows: Although I certainly am aware of all the wonderful benefits to be found in specially designed exercises to keep the body fit, I believe that even more wonderful benefits can be found through regular participation in active sports. Especially if one wants to look younger.

Notice that I say, specifically, *active* sports. Motorboating is a sport, but it will improve neither your mind nor your body. And I also do not mean hobby-type activities. Collecting stamps can be very rewarding, but it won't do a thing for flabby thighs.

What I mean, in this context, is a sport activity that gives you an unusual combination of benefits in three areas: physical, mental and social. This narrows the field down immediately to sports that are physically *and* mentally active and are usually performed farther away from home than your own bedroom. (That is not to eliminate the most wonderful sport of all, of course; love makes any woman younger.)

Sports such as swimming, jogging, bicycling, bowling, snow-skiing, water-skiing, horseback-riding, dancing (if the type of dancing you select requires mental effort), volleyball, golfing (without a golf cart), rowing, tennis, ice-skating, roller-skating—and I'm sure you can think of others— all require not only physical activity; they also require some degree of skill as well.

Let's look at the physical benefits first. They come to you in the form of both improved physical health and improved physical appearance. Active sports stimulate cardiovascular circulation; poor circulation is one of the chronic companions of age. They increase the strength of your muscles; muscular weakness is one of the first signs you are slowing down (as is witnessed by many women who feel a strain in their legs from simply climbing a long set of stairs). Physical exertion distributes the nutrients from your food, as mentioned briefly in chapter 2, thereby supplying your entire body with fuel. It helps you control your weight. It is self-evident, certainly, that most overweight people of both sexes are sedentary. If you know ahead of time that you have a sports engagement at a certain time of the day, I assure you, you'll think twice about overeating before you have to get up and move around with some vigor. The same result can be found in sports participation encouraging a lowered intake of alcohol (a great weight putter-onner). If you know at lunch that you have a four-o'clock tennis game, you'll be unlikely to have *two* glasses of wine. Aside from all of the above, regular sports activity increases your general energy level; it keeps you in a sort of physical-anticipation position that tends to focus your mind, even subconsciously, on activity, thus raising your awareness of the general life of your whole body.

Appearance is also improved through sports. Flabbiness becomes fiber as muscles tone their way to firmness. Women especially, with age, have a tendency toward loose thigh and buttock muscles. (And I don't mean *old* age; I mean thirty! Take an honest look.) The skin's appearance, and health, is improved as the blood is brought to the surface not only to feed and cleanse it, but also to leave a rosy glow of youth. And as you burn up calories, your weight will improve, making you look better (younger) as a bonus.

But the most beautiful bonus of active sports is that, unlike "exercise" exercising, which benefits primarily your body, you gain equal mental and psychological benefits from the exercise inherent in sports that require skill. Above all . . . pleasure. Not just the pleasure of movement, but the pleasure of accomplishment, of efficacy, of achievement. We all know that goals reached are a wonderful source of pleasure. Improving your skills in any sport will hand that pleasure to you on a regular basis, because each little improvement is a goal reached, and these goals come frequently as you progress in your abilities. It's not that you must be good at the sport to experience this pleasure; you only must be getting better. And that is assured if you engage in any sport on a regular basis.

This pleasure of achievement also brings mental peace and relaxation. As does the concentration required to perform any sport based on skill. Whether your tension and stress come from boredom or overwork or anxiety, total concentration with your mind on a particular, demanding stimulus will result in a newly refreshed mental attitude. And if you take lessons, you have the added stimulus of the learning experience. Young people are always learning; it feeds a curiosity, a progression of interest, a necessary excitement.

You may be thinking that you can achieve these mental benefits from activities such as bridge or chess, and you would be absolutely right. However, our emphasis in this chapter is on activities that specifically offer a youthful *appearance* to a woman, and active sports answer that aim to perfection via their physical activity. The mental boost, as I said, is a bonus (which, by the way, does its share in making you feel, hence look, younger).

Another bonus: You can augment, or vary, your social life through sports. And you wouldn't be the only one to want to stay young in this manner. Note the number of adult camps springing up all over the country. You can now take vacations learning to play tennis or ride horseback or just about whatever your sports-heart desires. But even if you take a "regular" vacation, you will not only enjoy yourself more, but you will also meet more people participating in a sport than you will reading in the sun and eating.

At home, too, you can enhance your social life. Sports partners, or even locker-room conversation, will offer you social contacts outside the normal work or family circles. Dates with men (even your husband) widen their appeal as you enjoy this kind of physical activity together, too, and then perhaps have a light meal together afterward.

After sports, there is nothing more relaxing or refreshing to both body and spirit than a steam bath and/or a massage. Youth pampers itself. You should, too. Health and beauty are both served. The warm water particles surrounding your entire body in a stream room promote circulation, hydrate your skin and soothe both your muscles and your nerves. A massage does the same for your circulation, muscles and nerves, moisturizes your skin and can become an occasional, special reward for taking care of yourself between massages. (It's another way, too, of keeping your weight down. I don't know a woman whose pride will let her take a massage if the condition of her body makes the procedure more like kneading dough.)

At this point, you should be saying, "Okay, I'm sold, but which active sport shall I choose?" And you stubborn ones will still be saying, "But I'm not athletic."

Be realistic. You cannot choose horseback-riding unless you have access to a horse. Look around your town to see what clubs and facilities are available. Money cannot become an excuse; I have yet to visit any town in America that does not have roads for bicycling, bowling alleys, high school tennis courts and a "Y" nearby that offers all sorts of activities and classes along with, usually, a swimming pool to boot. Consider not only availability but your own temperament. If you prefer to be alone and forego the social aspect of sports, you should not take up volleyball. If you're afraid of the water, swimming may not provide you with the right kind of pleasure. Simply use a little imagination and a lot of common sense; you *will* find a sport that's right for you if you try.

At last, if you are "not athletic," that does not mean you cannot participate in an active sport. You can learn. You can try. Saying "I'm *not* athletic" is like saying "I *don't* eat peas." It usually means you didn't when you were seven years old, but you haven't tried to reintroduce yourself to the thing since.

However, there can be valid reasons why you cannot participate in strenuous physical activity. For you, and only you, I will suggest walking and/or yoga. They both offer quite nice benefits if you give them a chance. Walking briskly for long distances (at least 30 minutes) will give your body exercise. Aside from that, it can provide time for contemplation and, as you note your surroundings, improve your powers of observation. Yoga gives mild physical exercise and does, although in a passive way, also provide mental relaxation in the sense that it utilizes concentration to some extent. I say "passive" because in yoga you do not actively exert your mental powers as you would in performing a skill. However, the very effort of concentrating on one single symbol for a period of time can release the mind from certain tensions simply by the very fact of distracting it from them during that time span.

Therefore, even if you are not athletic, you can become active in some sport and reap most of the benefits. If you are physically inclined, you have a wonderful new world opening up before you. And if you're already regularly active in an active sport, you are the one who can skip this chapter.

9
BECOMING YOUNG
... NOW

The major difference between people young in years and young people of any adult age is simply this: The chronologically young of our species acquire youth via an act of nature; an adult acquires youth via an act of will.

Both physically and mentally, up until the twenties or thirties, depending upon the individual, we are primarily receivers and processors; the first step into adulthood begins when we become, primarily, conceptualizers and creators—the most important thing to be created being our very selves, both physically and mentally. It is an interesting twist of human nature that, at a certain point, in order to succeed in continuing one's youth, one must first fulfill the requirements of becoming an adult. If an adult wishes to become young, now, it is no longer enough to continue *responding* to the outside world; one must *act* to create one's own world. It is the failure to make this crucial transition that results in such large numbers of "old" boys and girls— people of both sexes who are growing old physically while remaining immature mentally.

Our bodies up until that transition point into adulthood are a gift of our parents and Mother Nature; by their nature, they grow and shape themselves according to the programming of their genes. When Nature's function completes itself, it is up to the individual—now an adult physically—to maintain the finished product. If extra calories are consumed, the growing process will no longer utilize the fuel without any effort from you; you must put forth the energy to burn the calories as an act of conscious will, or carry the extra fuel, in the form of fat, around with you. Extra weight, in turn, because it results in a loss of energy, causes you to exercise less—which results in loss of strength and tone in the muscles—which results in not only flabbiness but also the inability to exercise easily—which results in even more excess fuel stored in the form of fat. And so the downward spiral of physical age continues, disuse leading progressively to degeneration. Once a body has reached its growth maturation, it must be used and maintained and cared for, just like any other product with working parts. One of the attributes of youth is physical energy in the forms of both growth and activity. Once adulthood has been reached, you can no longer exist, physically, on automatic pilot; growth has stopped (unless you are, unfortunately, growing outward), and activity has to be maintained manually.

The most paradoxical thing about many persons' aging habits is that at the very time they find themselves continuing to grow (improperly now) physically, they arrest the one growing process that is proper to man, which is, of course, mental growth. It is easy to grow mentally while still on the childhood side of the line marking adulthood. The surrounding world itself is wonderfully full of stimuli; parents, schools, peers, the physical and cultural worlds themselves are all there just bursting with things we don't know and want to learn. But at a certain point, we have received and processed most of what we need to know to take the next step—choosing for ourselves what input we need and desire to grow further mentally, in a direction we have chosen for ourselves. It is the lack of this direction, which must be conceptually and individually designed, that causes a great deal of mental aging. And even if the direction is chosen, you must still decide for yourself what new knowledge you need, what books must be read or classes taken or places visited. The completion of formal education, no matter at what level, is only the beginning of self-education, and you cannot get that by reading popular fiction, watching television and talking only with colleagues and friends. If one goes on passively, waiting to be spoon-fed what the world in general has to offer at a time when one should be *selecting* the input one needs for mental growth, then the results will, by necessity, be stagnation. And there is no such thing as stagnation in any living entity. A living thing is either growing and flourishing or dying.

Humans are luckier than all other living beings, however, because we can, through an act of will, continue the mental growth process the entire span of our lives; and we can, by the same kind of effort, maintain our bodies at some level of the flourishing stage even after its natural growth is completed.

But it takes effort.

The first effort to be made by any of us who wish not only to look younger but to continue our inner youth indefinitely, is to ask ourselves exactly what it is we're now missing that we think would not be missing if we looked or were in fact young . . . in years. The answer may be different for each of us, but there are a few choices to which you may add others or more applicable candidates of your own:

I would look or feel young again if I had:
My youthful body

Whatever body you now have, unless there is some health problem, can be returned, in principle, to the body of your young years. The question arises: Are you willing to put in the work and time required to regain that body? Most bodies go out of shape as they go out of condition, and it is true that a fit and shapely body is more youthful-looking than a flabby, unshapely one. If the physical appearance of your body is really the source of your problem, then do something about it. In America's culture today, more than at any other time and more than in any other country, the facilities available to you for reshaping or regaining your body are limitless. Diet doctors and clinics and books abound. Spas (more on this later), sprouting up from coast to coast, are devoted entirely to the purpose of reconditioning you from head to toe. Many companies, even, are providing gyms, running tracks and pools for employees who wish physical activity to use during lunch periods or after work. Exercise studios exist in every town for regular workouts.

Availability of facilities cannot be an excuse. And lack of money cannot be an excuse either—many places (like your local "Y") are within the financial reach of any American woman today. Therefore, if the shape and appearance of your body is *really* what you're missing . . . go get what you want.

I need not remind you that you cannot "get," through natural means, that which nature did not "give" you in potential, but any body can be beautiful and youthful if it is in prime condition and shape. However, if you decide—remember, the focus of this exercise is to consciously direct the course of your own life—that you are not willing to expend whatever effort is necessary (and *you* don't decide the amount of effort required, *reality* does) to attain or regain a fit and shapely body, then stop adding further to the aging process by expending the mental energy it takes to feel guilty or delve into self-pity or feel inferior because you do not have the body you wish to have. These forms of mental stress are probably more aging than all of the extra weight and bulges and knock-knees put together. Either change your body or make peace with yourself and go on living.

If, by the way, some particular part of your body is causing you mental anguish and it is something (like small breasts) that no amount of exercise can change, all is not lost. Once again, we live in an age when facilities and expertise are available to you. In certain cases, plastic surgery can be very helpful. In some cases, it can be less expensive than a psychiatrist who could help you properly out of the need for larger breasts (or whatever change you desire). But cosmetic surgery *is* available for otherwise unchangeable characteristics of your body that seem to be aging you. It is up to you; some effort will be required for any changes to be made, by you or a hired expert, in your bodily appearance.

I would look or feel young again if I had:
My youthful face

Because the face is exposed to all winds and weathers more than any other part of the body, it does show signs of aging sooner. These are not really signs of aging, but signs of living; however, in our particular culture it would be burying one's head in the sand not to recognize that, conventionally speaking, wrinkles and sags are negatively viewed by most Americans, men and women alike.

It's worth noting that America is the leader in this terribly demoralizing quest for the *appearance* of youth. In certain European countries, a woman isn't considered quite interesting until she's past forty. And in Europe, too, although women spend more time caring for themselves personally, they spend less time worrying about their actual age—caring for themselves not so much with the intention of looking younger, but in order to maintain themselves at their optimum level no matter what their chronological age. In America, women complain constantly (or suffer silently) about the signs of aging and do very little in the way of beneficial maintenance to retard these very signs. The tendency, here, is to try to shortcut the process and give the *appearance* of youth. This tendency is undoubtedly related to our parallel habits of attempting to *appear* to be wealthy, moral, sophisticated, etc., without ever discovering what those words mean.

In any event, if it is really a wrinkle-free, perfectly textured, moist and glowing facial appearance that would satisfy what you think is missing for you to feel a sense of youth, there are things that can be done. But you must *do* something. If the signs of aging are still superficial, the information given to you in chapters 2, 3, 4 and 5 should erase years in a matter of days. Proper skin care, proper nutrition, proper exercise and skillful makeup application will solve all but the most serious facial-structure flaws. But you must put forth the effort to cleanse your face properly morning and night (*never* going to bed wearing makeup), consciously control your food intake, decide on some form of regular exercise and take the time to practice makeup techniques. These things will not happen automatically; once across that line into adulthood, you have to make them happen.

If, as with the shape of your body, you have a structural characteristic that is causing you distress, much can be changed via cosmetic surgery. This, surely, should not become a catchall for solving problems, but is, today, a reasonable alternative. The most important factor in looking and feeling young is to gain confidence on the *inside*. If a large nose or a terribly lined and sagging facial appearance is what you're missing to make you look and feel younger, then by all means look into every possibility. But deal with the issue in some manner. Wishing will not make it so.

I would look or feel young again if I had:
Something important to look forward to

One of the most longed-for aspects of youth that adults are missing is that wonderful sense of tomorrow. And, further, that tomorrow will be important, that it could have in store some wonderful surprise or something new and exciting. Young people, in years, are always learning, expanding at least their knowledge if not their mental abilities. For some (erroneous) reason, many adults believe that at some given point in time—when they complete formal schooling or when they get married or establish a career or attain a certain financial level—they, as persons, are "finished." Once that attitude is adopted, aging sets in quite quickly because there can no longer be an inner sense of anticipation for the future. Given the limitless capacities of humans, we are *never* finished, and an undying youth results in great part from the joy of forward movement—forward to the new, the hoped-for, the tomorrows in life.

Youth follows a vision of what it will be. If you have already achieved the vision of your own youth, your vision was too limited. Create new visions, higher horizons. Learn and progress.

The stimulation of the learning process is never-ending. It creates internal youth in various ways. First, it gives one a sense of efficacy, of achievement; it can add to one's sense of self worth—not in the sense that achieving certain goals brings self-esteem but in the sense that lack of growth and lack of forward movement, when one is capable of it, can deplete one's sense of self-worth.

Personal progress is necessary in order to obtain the youthful excitement of goals set and won. Not vague goals like "I want to be happy," or "I want to look younger," but goals like "I want to finish my degree," "I want to go to work," "I want to learn to play bridge," "I want to get my body in shape" . . . goals that are specific and realistic enough to be achievable.

"Something important to look forward to" can be decided only by you, by you alone. Your husband's next business trip to San Francisco is not enough. It must be a goal of your own, worthy of your own capabilities, a goal that stretches you forward in some personal way.

When young people anticipate what they are going to "be" when they "grow up," they don't realize (and neither do most adults) even half of what they are saying. Because "being" is never over; there is always some way to "become" more. But you have to decide what more you wish to become.

If you wake up in the morning without any sense of anticipation for the day ahead, there is something wrong. Set about to right that wrong.

I would feel or look young again if I had:
A less hectic, more organized, more relaxed life

Poor organization, running here and there and running out of time, can honestly add years to anyone. The stress resulting from such turmoil is exhausting. One of the roads to feeling, hence looking, younger is to gain a greater control over your daily activities. Always arriving late for appointments, never managing to do all that you planned in one afternoon, wondering where the day went, all are signs of poor organization and usually an unrealistic sense of the whole issue of time as well.

This is not an uncommon problem for women and men alike in our fast-paced society. And it can be untangled. But, once again, it takes conscious effort. "Plan ahead" is the watchword here. And "don't plan too much." And "stop trying to *squeeze* extra things in between other activities." And "learn to say no."

In the morning, make a list—no, don't keep it all in your head; yes, you can, but why waste the energy when it isn't necessary?—of the things you would like to accomplish each day. Next, number the list in order of each activity's importance. Next, rewrite the list in order of location, with the most important activity leading the list. Now, how many hours do you think it will take to accomplish all of the things on your list including travel time? If a hectic schedule is wearing you down (and whom doesn't it wear down?), double the time you think it will take for each task. This is not just a method to slow you down; the truth is that, given all of the unexpected little incidents that happen in anyone's life each day, it will usually take twice as much time to accomplish your tasks as you think it will. The problem of overscheduling usually arises because most people plan their days as if everything will go like clockwork, and since *nothing* ever does, the schedule is already off by midmorning.

By utilizing the above method of scheduling, you will probably just manage to accomplish your reevaluated number of activities and nothing more, but you will do so with a sense of calm and control that will wipe lines of worry from your face day after day. And what would be so bad about having a little time left over to read the paper before everybody else dismembers all the sections?

If you're tempted to do something not on your list because you just happen to think of it or you're in the neighborhood, do it if you like, but strike something else from the list; in other words, substitute, but don't add. And, most importantly, if you have your day outlined and others ask you to do something for them or with them and you cannot rearrange other things in order to accommodate their request, say no. There is no other way around it; you just have to learn to be sweet but firm.

Aside from task accomplishment, the other major area that seems to bog women down or cause anxiety via the "I can't do it all" syndrome is the ability to keep up in the world of information input. This is a legitimate problem for everyone in our culture. The amount of information hurled at us daily from every corner is, objectively, mind-boggling.

There is only one way I know of to deal with this issue: the realization that you *can't* keep up with it all. And, really, there is no reason to try. But, again, decisions must be made.

In order to gain control over this problem, you must process information selectively. If the worlds of rock or disco music do not interest you, there is no need to be familiar with names of performers or progress(!) in those fields. On the other hand, if nutrition, as a subject, interests you, you will want to keep one ear open to hear any news in that area. Even via this method of exclusion, you will undoubtedly find yourself choosing to have interest in more areas than you would like from a processing point of view.

One means of organizing and finding time to keep up with information in your selected areas of interest is a filing system. I personally know many busy people (including myself) who employ this system with relative success. If you label filing folders with the subjects that interest you most, you immediately have a place for all of the articles you would like to read but do not have the time to do so at the moment you see them. When you come across such an article, simply clip it out and drop it into the proper file (this also eliminates stacks of magazines piled up to be read, which can be a formidable sight to anyone). Then, at another time, when you have a spare half-hour, you can open the file of your choice and read an article or two without any feeling of pressure. You can keep one miscellaneous file as well, for articles that are of some interest to you but not enough to warrant their own folder.

On a parallel subject, if there are television programs you would like to see but which cause a schedule conflict, a videotape recorder can be used very effectively to record and hold a show for you until you have the time to sit down and enjoy it.

If you have other pressured "hectic life" contexts, approach them in the same manner as the few suggestions offered here. Diffuse the pressure accompanying the task or subject by breaking it down into manageable bites and eliminate all areas that are not really important to your life.

I would feel or look young again if I had:
Time for myself

How many minutes a day do you spend either on the telephone or watching television or visiting with friends? These are three of the greatest time consumers that cause women, especially, to claim that they have no time for themselves. You cannot spend *that* much time at the office or cleaning house, no matter how demanding your work or how large your home (and children are the greatest excuse for laziness in the world). In order to become young as an adult, you must regain some of the selfishness you had when you were, in fact, a youth. Youth pampers itself; it exhibits a sense of self-importance that, unfortunately, many adults relinquish in the face of grown-up responsibilities.

I once had a woman tell me that when her bedroom door was closed— the bedroom being her place to hide away to think or work toward some goal or simply pamper herself with a bubble bath in the adjoining bathroom—the rest of her family knew that she was not to be disturbed except in an emergency. Another told me, with some wry amusement, that when she did not want to be approached or disturbed, she wore a particular hat around the house, which meant that she wanted to be alone with herself. Amusing, perhaps, but it worked for her.

There are many reasons to demand from your family the time and consideration for your own, private life. First, *you* need it. Everyone needs time to devote exclusively to his or her own needs, whatever those needs may be. Nonstop distraction or activities involving others encourages lack of attention to oneself and one's personal requirements for private endeavors or enjoyments. Especially if you have a family, it is very easy to lose a sense of yourself and your own youthful feelings by devoting yourself to the service and the needs of others. Serve yourself as well.

Surprisingly enough, you will undoubtedly do your family a service in the process; by teaching them to respect your needs for time to yourself, they may learn to rely on themselves much more and perhaps grow into more responsible adults through such awareness. On the other hand, if you are using your family's and friends' needs or desires to help you evade the decision making that you yourself require, then you do not have a *time* problem.

Apart from all the mental and psychological benefits to be gained from creating a private, personal life for yourself, there are many external, beauty benefits as well. And, yes, they can most assuredly make you lose years in appearance along with their other obvious, internal benefits. Daily skin care, regular exercise or sports activity, makeup application, wardrobe expansion and/or alteration, books to be read, classes to attend, careers to be pursued—things from which you directly benefit—all contribute their share in making you young . . . now.

Special "Pampering Yourself" Treats

GOING TO A SPA

Special spas are an ever-growing phenomenon in our country, and although they are expensive, they can be a wonderful way to pamper yourself. (You will note that, as they become more popular, many are being formed that are less expensive as well.) Spas can also perform the function of acting as a launching pad to start you on your way back to a youthful way of living and caring for yourself.

The level of seriousness is different at the various spas, and you should determine which one you wish to visit upon the basis of this difference. At some of them, when you check in, you are expected to follow precisely the exercise and diet regimes prescribed for you. At others, classes and facilities and fixed-calorie diets are available and you determine yourself what kind of regime you will follow. If pampering is your purpose, you would want the latter; that way you can exercise just enough to make you feel good (preventing sore muscles) and spend the rest of your time taking steambaths, massages, facials, herbal wraps, hand and foot care, makeup lessons, etc. (You will be *shocked*—as you will, I hope by following the ten-day program in this book—at how much better and younger you can look by spending one week at a spa where you have nothing to do but devote time and energy to yourself.) If, on the other hand, you want to begin a serious program to "get your act together," you will want a strict environment in order to accomplish as much as you can in the short amount of time you will stay at the spa.

One of the side benefits of going to a spa is that you will meet other women from all over the country who are there for the same purposes you are. There is a wonderful sense of camaraderie that can act very positively in helping you gain the enthusiasm you need to change your way of living.

The one trap you must not fall into—and the same trap waits for you at the end of this present ten-day program—is slipping back into old habits once you return home. It's very easy to care for yourself and devote time to yourself when each activity is planned for you and/or there is nothing else to do. When the spa—or the program—is behind you, then those first few days afterward are when you *must* make the effort *yourself* to keep going, keep that youthful behavior and make it a way of life. If you don't, there is not a soul in the world who can help you, and you will have only yourself to blame. In the end, it is you who must make the efforts.

CREATING A "SPA" IN YOUR OWN HOME

You can—alone or with other women—create a wonderful spa right in your own home (or someone else's who has the room). If there is an extra room, or an attic or basement that is not being used, you can turn that room into a most inspiring spa in which to pamper yourself and/or a haven at which to meet friends for the same purpose. The decor is important; it should be feminine with lots of luxurious touches—this need not cost a great deal of money, it just takes a little imagination. There should be a lounge chair for reading, magazines for browsing, a makeup table for experimenting, facilities (hot plate or professional vaporizer) for giving facials. . . . You can take the idea as far as your desires and pocketbook will permit: a massage table, exercise equipment (there are gadgets that will stablize a regular "road" bicycle for exercising purposes), sinks and/or shower, steam room or cabinet. It can be a place for you to hide away and renew yourself or a special, relaxed atmosphere for friends to gather or drop in at will. You can give each other facials, compare notes on fashions and current events in the manner of a permanent beauty spa or club. I assure you, alone or with others, such a spot, always ready and waiting for you, will encourage you to stay young after you become young again.

THE PROVERBIAL BUBBLE BATH

The idea of an evening in the bath is as old as Rome; the only wonder is that more women do not partake of its benefits. If your bathroom is designed only for function, you are missing a great deal indeed. Beautiful surroundings are soothing, especially in a room where one's beauty is maintained. Pretty towels, bottles, carpeting, fresh flowers, plants—all lovely and feminine touches—act to remind a woman that she is a *woman*, too, not just a person.

In order to get the most out of an evening bubble bath—unless the man in your life wishes to join you; then you get to pamper each other—set yourself up properly and make sure you will not be interrupted (do not permit your children to dominate your life to the extent that you cannot spend two hours alone in the bath!).

You will need:

• a good book or a magazine or pencil and pad for jotting down notes (or none of these if you wish simply to relax and contemplate)

• several big, pretty towels laid out and waiting for you

• a pretty carafe, filled with either mineral water or white wine or juice or a soft drink, sitting on a small table beside the tub (preferably in an ice bucket to keep it cold—this is very refreshing while sitting in a warm bath)

• beauty mask ingredients premade into a mask if you wish to give yourself a facial as well

• a perfumed beauty soap (your regular deodorant soap does not exactly add to a pampering atmosphere)

• your favorite perfume in the following forms: bubble bath or bath oil, powder and cologne or toilet water

• one bottle sesame (or other vegetable) oil—can be scented with perfume or bath oil

• a pumice stone (for polishing elbows, heels, etc., free of callouses) if necessary

• manicuring equipment if you wish to do your nails while in the bath

• a lovely robe (not your morning housecoat) and slippers

How you will actually *take* the bath must be left up to you. Some women find the action of manicuring and/or beauty masks a method of pampering; others find it distracting. The addition of a Jacuzzi attachment to your tub can give you the added feature of a whirlpool. However, if you simply roll up a towel and place it behind your head—or use a bath pillow—it can be exquisite to do nothing at all in your bath except just lie back, sip on something cool and let the warmth and sweet smells from the water itself relax both your muscles and your mind.

After the bath, step out onto something soft and fluffy and dry yourself leisurely with one of those pretty towels. If you have washed your hair, use another to wrap around your head and keep your wet hair away from your face. Next, smooth the oil over your entire body in small amounts so that you feel sleek and silky. While the oil is penetrating the skin of your body, finish your facial cleansing with skin freshener and apply your moisturizing or protection cream. Now, fluff your perfumed bath powder all over your body and slip into your pretty robe and slippers. Comb or brush your hair and add a top layer of scent with your cologne or toilet water, patting or spraying some of it into your hair as well. Cream your hands well and add, if you like, a touch of color to your lips and cheeks (you can remove it again just before bed).

This is a pampering evening you can give yourself as often as you like. Everybody has a bathtub; so time, money, etc., cannot be excuses. Do it for yourself once in a while; you may just like it.

A PROFESSIONAL MASSAGE, FACIAL, MANICURE OR PEDICURE

From time to time, every woman should pamper herself with one of the above, even if only once a year. Don't say you can't afford it that infrequently, not if you could afford this book. All of these things can be done at home by yourself, of course—instructions for all of them are given in these chapters (except for the massage, and I'm sure the man in your life can figure that one out)—but there is really nothing as pampering as to have them done for you. The relaxed feeling of just lying back and letting someone else do the work is unbeatable. Even if you have never tried it before, try it soon. Most good department stores have beauty salons where you can get all but the massage, as do many hairdressing salons. For the massage, most "Y's" have a resident masseuse, as do all health clubs; you can also find licensed masseuses in the phone book who will come to your home. Many hotels offer all of these services, so if there is one in your town, you can simply go there. But wherever or whenever, let a professional pamper you once in a while; it's worth it.

TAKING A WEEKEND VACATION—ALONE

One of the factors contributing to the sense of a lack of youth that many women feel is the lack of time spent alone. This is understandable and has been treated, to some extent, earlier in this chapter. If you feel a loss of yourself because of schedules, family or whatever, taking a minivacation alone can be a wonderfully renewing way not only of pampering yourself but getting in touch with yourself as well.

Especially for women who do not have the independence of work or a career, it can be an exhilarating experience. Drive or fly or take a bus to a place near or far, depending upon both your nerve and/or pocketbook. Make your travel plans by yourself or with the help of a travel agent— *not* your husband. If you feel nervous about checking in at airports or hotels, make *sure* to exercise this method of pampering yourself—you need it for your own sense of independence.

Depending upon the place you have chosen to go, plan your general activity ahead of time. If you are visiting a big city from a small one, you may want to go shopping, or to some cultural event, or to a special restaurant. If you are going to a country hotel or a friend's cabin, you may just want to take along a good book and walking shoes for a very contemplative few days.

What you do and where you go are not nearly so important as doing it and going it *alone*. You may wish you had a friend along, or the man in your life, but believe me, in the end you will feel refreshed and more energetic than when you left. Not only will you have time to yourself for introspection, but just the simple fact of handling all of the things that will come up *by yourself* will give you a wonderful feeling of *you* as a person. It may be difficult to get yourself going on this particular venture, but once you see how rewarding it can be, I think you'll agree that it is, in fact, a wonderful way to pamper yourself.

I'm sure you will be able to come up with many more exciting or relaxing methods of pampering; but be sure to do *something* for yourself —and for you alone—once in a while. The lift it will offer you mentally and the relaxation it will offer you physically will both add to your life and subtract from your years.

10

FINGERTIPS TO TOES

It needs to be written down simply somewhere. It may as well be here. Manicures and pedicures are easy, timeless procedures *not* involving a hundred steps. Learn to do them quickly and efficiently as a mere maintenance routine, and then just do them regularly and forget about any worries—whether or not to cut cuticles or file in one direction or buff or not buff, etc. The only fun comes in choosing colors of polish anyway.

Manicures

How to Give Yourself a Manicure

1. Remove all old polish and wash and dry hands.

2. File nails with a fresh emery board until you have the desired shape. The best way to determine the shape is to observe the size and roundness of the base of the nail where the cuticle is attached. Generally speaking, if you file the end of the nail to match the base oval, you will achieve a well-proportioned, natural-looking nail. Pointed ends or flat ends are very artificial in appearance. The choice of shape, however, is up to you. As far as length is concerned, the most attractive, natural look is approximately one-third longer than the rest of the nail. In filing, do not "saw" at your nails. Whatever direction seems easiest

for you (or both) is the one to follow, but make your strokes with the file rather long and decisive. Make sure you do not leave any rough edges.

3. Pour some steel-ground oatmeal (the same kind you use for a defoliating facial), which you have pulverized in your blender, into a large bowl and set it next to the sink.

4. Fill the sink with warm, soapy water and soak your hands until the cuticles are soft. (While your hands are submerged, you can use a nail-white pencil under your nails to be sure they are clean.) Next, with a cuticle pusher or another nail, gently push back the cuticle on each finger. If your cuticles are small, this may be enough. If they tend to grow large over your finger, when you push them back, they may be too obvious. In the latter case, you can trim them with cuticle scissors, which are available in any drugstore. If you trim them, be sure you don't leave any ragged ends (this could cause a hangnail—which is why most experts recommend against it—but if you're careful, it can give a more finished look).

5. "Wash" wet hands with the oatmeal—over and over—in order to remove any dead skin cells from the skin of your hands and give them a smooth, young appearance.

6. Dry hands and cream them. Leave them "virgin" for several hours (overnight, if possible) so that the nails can breathe naturally, and then wash again and apply polish.

Applying Nail Polish

1. Apply a clear undercoat. This protects the nail and keeps it from discoloration, which can result from applying color directly to the nail. If your nails are weak, your undercoat should be some form of nail hardener. Let dry completely.

2. Apply color polish of your choice. Unless you plan to change your nail color with a change of clothes, I recommend selecting a color that either matches or harmonizes with your basic makeup palette color for everyday wear. Remember that dark colors draw attention, so if the skin on your hands shows its age, lean toward subtle, medium shades that will enhance your hands without focusing on them. Apply one or two coats and let dry completely.

3. Apply a clear outer coat or sealer. This adds shine to your finished nails as well as protecting the nail color from chipping so easily. If your nails are weak, this outer coat should be some form of nail hardener.

Tips

1. If your nails are weak, bring each coat of clear polish over the end and under the tip of each nail. This will help to strengthen the nail.

2. If your nails are weak, be sure you are eating enough protein and try taking gelatin capsules, or dissolve one packet of gelatin powder in a glass of juice each day.

3. During the week or ten days between full manicures, paint new coats of color and outer coat right over the old polish if it chips. Nothing ruins the looks of a hand more than chipped nail polish.

4. If you need to dry your nails in a hurry, use your blow-dryer or plunge your hands into ice water.

5. Do not dial the telephone with your finger. Use a pencil or some such instrument.

6. If you soak your hands in warm olive oil once or twice a week it will soften the appearance of your hands and strengthen your nails. (If you can go to bed afterward, without removing the oil and wearing a pair of white cotton gloves, all the better.)

7. Anything that increases circulation aids in stimulating nail growth —even just pinching the ends of the fingers.

Pedicures

Pedicures are, in principle, just like manicures. The only difference is in shaping. It is best to cut toenails straight across (perhaps rounding just a bit at the corners) and then file to ensure that there are no rough edges. This simple shape is the safest for hose, which can be torn by any points on toenails, and it looks much more attractive anyway.

(Both manicures and pedicures can be done while taking a luxurious bubble bath, by the way. Everything gets soaked properly while *you* are enjoying the relaxation and pampering of a lovely bath. Don't forget the oatmeal treatment for your feet as well as your hands, and don't worry about the oatmeal getting into your bath water; it acts as a softening agent for all of your skin.)

Polish for toenails is applied in the same order and manner as for fingernails, and my personal taste calls for matching colors, but that is certainly an optional issue. The only helpful addition might be to place a cotton ball or two between each toe so that they will be spread wide enough not to smudge each other's polish.

And that's it. Not the most important subject in the world, but very important for an overall look of youth and good grooming.

11
CREATING A PERSONAL LIFE-STYLE

As you may have gathered, the underlying theme of this entire book is to help you get to know, get to like and individualize your own individuality. You have only one life to lead. That platitude, I know, is so overworked that it is certain to sound trite. But triteness does not invalidate truth. Very few people on this earth ever really identify who they are, what they are doing and why. Those who do—who "live" their one life—have discovered the only possible fountain of youth.

Anyone can. But it takes thought and effort, the same kind you have been making for the past many days. Now you can expand much of your new knowledge about yourself into other parts of your life as well. First identify who you are and what you want. Then look at reality. Then make the two match. Not *literally* match—which is the mistake most people make when they try to do this—but match in *principle*. If I make it sound easy, it isn't. But it is possible and it is necessary if you wish to bring into existence the life-style you could be living. Now.

Life-styles usually fall into two categories: conventional and rebellious. "Conventional," of course, means that the life-style was never consciously developed; that it has been acquired by randomly and uncritically (or emotionally) picking up ideas, values and ways of living that are more or less "in the air" (meaning coming your way via friends,

174

family, television, etc.). Most people who lead conventional lives do so because they have failed to think independently and have never decided conceptually what type of life they would like to lead. Living a conventional life is, of course, much easier than examining or creating a personally designed life, but it is also, by its very passive nature, less fulfilling as well.

On the other side, most people who attempt to lead an *un*conventional life end up merely rebelling against conventionality. Rather than take the time and effort required to learn what must be learned about themselves (and created by themselves) in order to be truly unconventional— which means original—they rush to join any one of a variety of so-called unconventional groups or causes or modes of dress or life-styles that *proclaim* themselves unconventional. By doing this, they merely end up conforming to the accepted standards (or conventions) of some new group instead of the group from which they are fleeing.

A *personal*, unconventional life-style is not substituting one group's conventions for another. It is not, in fact, a group action of any sort at all. It is not, in other words, *not* conforming to anyone else's standards. It is setting standards of your own. Consciously developing a personal life-style is the only way to acquire an individual, truly unconventional mode of living. It is a positive act, *against* nothing and no one. It is an act of love. Toward oneself . . . and one's own life.

And, as mentioned earlier, it is not necessarily easy.

But it *is* incomparably and endlessly fascinating. It is full of wonder and unexpected surprises. It is a most exhilarating adventure.

And it will keep you young. The young don't *settle*.

In order to lead a personal, thoughtful life, at any age, one must first decide to think. One can hardly expect to develop an individual life-style if one relinquishes one's own mind to the changing winds of mass input from others.

Next decision. What to think about? Important subjects come immediately to mind: work, mate, friends and family, house, leisure time . . . This one chapter, obviously, will not—and cannot—provide answers. But it can provide a blueprint, a methodology, by which you can discover your own answers.

Jobs Are More Than Money (Maybe)

Is money a major value to you? No? Fine. Yes? Fine. As long as your answer is your own honest answer. But if money is a major value to you and there is no future possibility of great financial advancement in your present job, you may want to consider changing to another type of work that you might not even enjoy as much, but which has greater potential for earnings. If pleasure in your work is more important to you than earnings received, know this consciously and be happy that you have fulfilled your major goal.

Another question to ask yourself about work: Do you hold the conventional opinion that work—by definition—is something one *has* to do and that it is usually an unpleasant task? Work can and should be largely an enjoyable experience. If yours is not, think about what kind of work would be enjoyable. Consider this question without any thought as to whether or not it is possible given your particular context or educational background. Just answer the question, What would I like to do, pie-in-the-sky dreaming like to do?

Only unhampered thinking of this nature can give you access to your inner mind. Write down a list of anything that comes to mind. Next, rearrange the list in order of preference.

Now and only now, consider reality. Are you qualified to pursue anything in this area of work? Are you located so that work of this nature is within reach? Are you willing to work the amount of hours such a job would require? Would you really like to work in this field *every* day? Do you have a realistic idea of what this kind of work really entails, or are you glamorizing it? Do you really like best to work with people, or would you prefer working with animals, or machines, or ideas?

The answers to questions such as these can be quite surprising if you have never consciously considered them before. Even if you have, perhaps the answers have changed as you have developed along your own personal growth pattern.

If the work you are now doing does not satisfy your major value goals, consider how you can alter it or change it completely. It doesn't matter if you are fifty—you only have one life. If you feel an entirely new field would be best for you, consider how you can begin to make the change —further education, move, etc.—and, most importantly, if you decide that you would rather not make the efforts required, or that other, higher values (like staying in a town where your children are going to college, or having the free time to travel with your husband) prevent it, know that this, too, is a conscious decision, that you have dealt with your priorities honestly, and have peace of mind that given all considerations, you *are* doing what you would like to do.

Mating Is Not a Game . . .

. . . and opposites do not attract. Another conventional value you are holding? Do they? Maybe they do. Maybe not? Only you can decide what you think about those statements.

A romantic relationship is without doubt the most important of all relationships—and sex is *not* hamburger. Somewhere deep inside each of us, we know this. If your behavior does not reflect your true values on the subject, whom are you hurting?

In order to determine your own value system, you must question church and community alike, parents and most of history, taboos and fears . . . but romantic relationships can be examined by exactly the same method in which you dealt with employment—by rationally and honestly determining your own hierarchy of values. It does no good to stick your head farther into the sand; your unhappiness or frustration or uncertainty will go right on aging you whether or not you consciously confront it.

Write down a list of all of the attributes you admire in a man. Rearrange them in order of importance. This is not a marriage manual, but if your own husband or love partner does not exhibit those characteristics, it is worth some thought. Perhaps you have never told him these things are important to you. Perhaps you never knew yourself.

The point I am trying to make here is this: Your own personal love life requires conscious thought and conscious effort. I think nothing ages a person faster than personal unhappiness in the romantic area of life. Set about getting yours in order if it is not.

Families—The Unchosen People

This is a very heavily discussed subject of late. Is marriage obsolete? Is the family nucleus breaking up? Does divorce scar people for life?

Have you caught the error? All of these subjects are approached in the "collective" form. These questions, discussed this way, deal with the norm. How do these things affect most people? Your goal is not to care, unless the information can help you in making your own decisions. Poll-taking can never help *you* make up *your* mind.

The questions you must ask are, Is marriage obsolete for me? Would divorce be an advantage for me? Or not? The question is *not*, Is it OK not to love one's parents? The question *is*, do you love yours?

Of all of the things with which you must interact in this life, the one with which you have the greatest number of options is the people with whom you choose to interact. Relatives are no exception, unless you have taken the responsibility of bringing a child into the world. But even children require the same judgment as adults, relatives or not. You can love them, or not. You can see them, or not (after they're adults). You can put up with their behavior, or not. Always examining the consequences of your decisions and being able to live with those consequences, you may establish your value system concerning your family with the same consciousness as you do other, albeit less emotional, subjects.

The most important consideration to eliminate in order to determine your real values concerning people is duty or obligation. If you have children, for example, it is your responsibility to care for them until they reach a certain age, but it is not your duty to have any more. Suppose, if you are honest with yourself, you decide that you really wish you had never borne children in the first place. Nothing is sacrilegious to *think* about if it is honest. If you come to such a decision, it doesn't mean you don't love your present children or enjoy them now; it may mean you should not only not bear more, but that you should also begin now to prepare for the life you would prefer to live the moment they are no longer your responsibility. You can go to school while they are in school, and you can begin getting involved in your preferred interest area on some level sooner than you think.

The point here is to *think* about your family and friendships. If you don't really enjoy certain company, start cutting down the amount of time you spend with that company. If you have permitted others too much intimacy into your life, start retraining them as to how close you wish them to be. But before you do any of this, you must decide consciously what you want and do not want.

Finding the "Life" in Life-style

At last, in the personal expressions of your own individuality, are you living your own life? Many people believe (wrongly) that they cannot live the way they want to because they don't have enough money. This is absolutely false.

That is not to say that, at some point, money does not enter into the picture. But it *is* to say that it is not a primary in devising a life-style that fulfills your needs and desires. Not today. And not in America.

Once again, it is a matter of thinking in principle before acting in fact.

In Principle:

1. Approach each subject as if money were not an issue. This will allow you to assess *honestly* what you would really like. The first question should be, What do I want?

2. Eliminate any considerations of duty or obligation.

3. Ask if the situation *can* be changed (if you have arthritis, you may not be able to play handball, etc.).

4. Determine how you can get as close to what you want *stylistically*. (This is the key to enjoyment—if the *quality* of what you want is present, you will feel that your own personal life-style has been achieved. *Quantity* is only a degree.)

YOUR HOME

Using the above guideline, what kind of home would you really like? This is important; a home is an important personal statement. Don't just decide on a certain kind of home or a certain neighborhood because that is what you think you can afford. You can have, in principle, any kind of home you choose. Decide which considerations are most important to you. Write out a list and rearrange the items in order of preference. City or country living? Modern or traditional? Large or small? Isolated or neighborly? You can adjust the size or the amount, but at least achieve your major preferences. If you want a big, traditional home in the country and you are living in a ranch-style surrounded by other ranch-styles, think about how you can adjust your context at least to get to the country if that is the most important. You might find you would be happier in a charming old farmhouse in the countryside than packed together in a new, small house on a sidewalked street. Or if the reverse is true, you might be happier packed into a small apartment, but able to enjoy the cultural life of a city. *Think* about it. If you have a family, sit down with everybody and think together about it. Don't settle.

YOUR CAR

Want a Ferrari? Don't drive a Chevrolet. Get some form of sportscar, whatever *you* can afford (or get a used car). You will always feel a special rush of youth when you get into a car that expresses your own style. If you want a luxury car, get the top of the line in a less expensive make, but get the *best* of what you can afford.

LEISURE TIME

This is the easiest of all to alter in order to express your individual style. What do you *want* to do? If you want to go to Europe and can't afford it, go to Old Quebec City. If you want to go to the Bahamas and can't afford a winter vacation there, wait and go off-season. If you want a big boat on the ocean, get a big boat on a lake or a little boat on the ocean; if you want a vacation alone without the kids and you can't afford to go away, send the kids away. There are a million ways to alter leisure time to achieve the experience of doing what you want to do, but you must use a little imagination. Going to relatives for a week to save hotel bills and wishing you were alone the whole time may be not much cheaper and a lot less satisfying than staying alone together at a local hotel for the weekend. *Think* before you travel.

ENTERTAINING

This above all subjects does not take sums of money. Most parties are boring because they are not planned, and it therefore *seems* that lavish food is the most important element only because it offers the only real difference in parties. What you serve is not nearly so important as what you do and who is there. Give thought to your guest list—people are interesting to people. Theme parties can be enormously successful. Food, the only really expensive item for a party, is the least important ingredient. Entertaining at home and going out, too, should be given thought. If you like to dine at lavish restaurants, go out seldom, but go out the way you want to.

Enough said. I'm sure you get the idea by now. Youth is promise. Youth looks to the future, and is not afraid of change. If you want something more and want to become something more, it is very likely that you are in need of only one ingredient: you. As you are now. Not as you were twenty years ago, or ten years ago, or last year. Now.

Recapturing a lost youth is not the answer. Creating a present youth means becoming young now . . . and "young" means curiosity, it means searching, it means achieving a vision of yourself and your life that is you. It means shedding all of that unconsciously accumulated baggage— all of those "accepted" standards—that you do not choose to carry, retaining, of course, those with which you decide to agree. It means establishing (though your own effort) standards and values and actions that will result in your own happiness.

Somewhere deep inside each of us, we know that we are unique, that we are unrepeatable, that we are an original. The key to realizing in actuality this inner knowledge, I submit, is understanding that these attributes are not givens at birth, but that they are potentials. They are possibilities. It becomes our responsibility, then—each one of us, alone and by ourselves—to give form and shape consciously to these possibilities. In this manner, we may live out and express our uniqueness, therefore exciting our own lives, as well as others, with our individuality.

If our minds are free to open honestly not only to the outside world but also to our inner truths, our eyes might just perceive some part of life in a little different light, our brains might think of some unexpected thought, or our imaginations dream up some lovely new pleasure. These, after all, are the hallmarks of youth, the great joys of being human . . . and of being beautiful at any age.

12

OVER THIRTY-FIVE: QUESTIONS AND ANSWERS

When I speak at women's clubs, town hall celebrity series or fund raisers, there is usually a question-and-answer period following the lecture. I have compiled here a list of the most frequently repeated questions and their answers. Interestingly enough, many of the same questions pop up all over the country. Since they are so commonly asked, some of these answers may touch on subjects that have been plaguing you as well.

On Skin

Q. How do you feel about protein supplements for the skin?

A. Protein is one of the few things that can benefit your skin both from the inside and the outside. Good nutrition, rich in protein, is necessary for the health of your skin, but protein in the form of a good beauty mask (like the whipped yolk of an egg) can help to repair some surface damage of the skin as well, thereby improving its appearance from the outside.

Q. Does foundation makeup protect the skin?

A. If foundation is applied over a properly cleansed and moisturized or protected facial skin, it can act as a further barrier between the skin and such pollutants as city air and other makeup. I know women in New York who wouldn't leave the apartment without foundation for just this reason.

Q. Is it true that cod liver oil is good for the skin?

A. It is certainly good for it from the inside; cod liver oil is rich in vitamins A and D, both essential for the health of your skin. As far as application on the surface of the skin is concerned, it is unlikely that it can have an appreciable effect; remember that the skin is able to absorb vitamins from the outside in, in minute quantities only. Some success has been achieved by the external application of vitamin A for acne victims, but for a normally healthy skin, I don't imagine it would make that much difference because of the above-mentioned reason.

Q. Is there any way, other than plastic surgery, to get rid of lines around the mouth and eyes?

A. Yes. Dermabrasion or chemical peels or silicone injections are all possible methods; however, as with cosmetic surgery, you must research the subject carefully and select a doctor with even greater care; there is no cure-all for the permanent elimination of lines and wrinkles, and there is risk involved in any of the present methods. Know what you are doing and go at the subject slowly.

Q. What about temporary line tighteners?

A. Care must be exercised with any of these products, including natural ones like egg whites, that they do not further stretch and dry the skin. I would suggest using them only after correspondence with the manufacturer or a discussion with a dermatologist as to the ingredients in the product. Also, be aware that although you may look wonderful at the beginning of an evening wearing such a temporary tightener, they *are* temporary; if it's to be a late evening, you may find your face falling before your very eyes.

Q. I have heard that smoking can cause little vertical lines around the mouth. Is this true?

A. Absolutely. The sucking action of smoking, if you do it on a regular basis, puckers the mouth repeatedly with each inhalation, which can lead to the formation of many lines, early.

Q. What can I do for puffiness under the eyes when I wake up in the morning?

A. One method of preventing puffiness, which is often nothing more than water retention, is to sleep on two pillows instead of one; this keeps the head at an angle that prevents the water from accumulating. Another method is the application of cold, wet tea bags to the eyes and lying back down for ten minutes. Some women swear by the application of grated potato, but I cannot personally do so—tea bags work well and are so much easier.

Q. Is it true that the aloe vera plant is good for sunburns?

A. Yes. And for any type of superficial burn. I always recommend keeping an aloe plant in the kitchen. Then, if you burn yourself, you can quickly run the burn under cold water, break a leaf in two and apply the gel before any swelling occurs. The gel from the aloe is also a good beauty mask for dry and aging skins.

Q. I am thirty-six, but I still get breakouts on my skin like a teenager; what is going on?

A. This is not as uncommon as you may think. Some dermatologists call this phenomenon "secondary adolescence acne." Even if it is only an occasional problem, it usually is brought on by an overactivity on the part of the sebaceous glands, which can be stimulated by many things, including improper diet, but which dermatologists usually pinpoint to stress. If this condition is anything other than occasional—in which case you treat it to perfect hygiene and drying agents—you should see a dermatologist for specific diagnosis and treatment. (A good beauty mask for troubled areas is fresh tomato juice and dried mint leaves.)

On Hair

Q. What can I do for split ends?

A. Condition your hair with both protein and cream conditioners every time you wash it. Cutting the hair often, snipping off the damaged ends, will eliminate the problem; but if you wish to let your hair grow longer, most hair treatment centers offer "singeing," which will seal the ends for a rather long period of time.

Q. Can you safely perm fine hair?

A. The answer is "No, but . . ." meaning that, generally speaking, the results will be very dissatisfactory, but if your hairdresser is extremely knowledgeable and careful, it *can* be done. A minute or two either way can make the difference, though, so it's all in the hands of the operator.

Q. Can I perm color-treated hair?

A. The answer here is "Yes, but . . ." meaning that, generally speaking, one should not subject the hair to two chemicals. However, if neither the coloring or the perming is overdone, it can be done. The same is true for hair straightening.

Q. What is a good conditioning treatment for dry, damaged hair?

A. Most commercial protein treatments (not conditioners) will help to temporarily correct the damage, but the easiest, and often most beneficial, treatment is the simple application of pure, virgin olive oil (found in the health food store). Wash and rinse hair well, next towel-dry gently until most of the water is out of your hair but it is still wet. Heat ½ cup of olive oil until very warm and rub gently into hair (staying away from the scalp if it is naturally oily). Now, wrap hair tightly with a thin towel that has been thoroughly soaked in hot water—do not wring out until "dry." Next, either wrap again with another towel or sit under a hair-dryer on "hot" for ten minutes (be sure no water touches any electrical connection), then rewash hair and finish with a cream conditioner. When hair is completely dry, you may wish to brush a *very small amount* of the olive oil through the bulk of your hair to tame it and give it a lovely shine—don't use too much or it will look stringy and attract dust.

Q. My hair is very fragile: How can I keep it from breaking into many different lengths?

A. Do not use electric rollers or sit under a hair-dryer or use a blow-dryer any more often than you absolutely have to. All three will damage fragile hair. Also, do not rub your hair with a towel after washing; merely *press* the water out of your hair.

Q. I am fifty-two years old and love long hair, but everybody keeps saying that it ages a woman, What should I do?

A. You should, first of all, look around at several very well-known women just about your age who wear long hair and look wonderful. It is not your age that determines the length of your hair; it is your face shape (*and* condition), your body shape(*and* condition), your life-style and your personality style. If you are a long-hair person on the "inside," you should, by all means, wear your hair in a style with some length. The style and length ("long" meaning no longer than shoulder-length) will be determined by the above factors, and you should always remember to keep the style soft.

Q. I know you don't like gray hair, but I am sixty years old with silver-white hair. Do you think there's anything wrong with that at my age?

A. The answer is, "Yes, unless . . ." meaning that, generally speaking, gray or white or silver or any combination of the preceding ages a person terribly. However, if you have a flair for the dramatic that will offset normal connotations of this color hair *or* if you exhibit such character stature that the older but "queenly" look only adds to the esteem you elicit from others, you may be able to carry it off. But not many can.

On Diet and Exercise

Q. Do you have any exercise that will firm jowls?

A. Sit straight and tip your head back as far as you can (you will feel your neck muscles pulling, which will also firm your neck and under-chin areas). Now, open your mouth into a smile (making sure not to squint your eyes and deepen lines there) and jut the lower lip out and up, not losing the smile. Relax jaw and repeat six times each day.

Q. What do you think of jogging?

A. It is an excellent body conditioner *if* done properly—proper shoes, properly fitted, running on a track. Experts in this field of running warn continually against running on concrete in normal sneakers—bone damage can show up years later—but people the country over don't seem to hear them.

Q. What do you think of jumping rope as an exercise?

A. Very good, and portable, too. Jumping on carpet or earth is easier on your feet and leg bones than concrete.

Q. What do you, personally, do when you need to lose a couple of pounds fast?

A. I eat a baked potato and fried eggs for dinner. The potato, being carbohydrate, fills you up (and one medium potato is only around 100 calories), and the eggs, being protein, stick with you. And it's delicious. I bake the potato in foil (no oil) and fry two eggs (using a vegetable oil spray), then just split the potato and slip the soft eggs inside. A little salt and pepper and you feel as if you are splurging instead of dieting and you're only consuming 250 calories. During the day, I nibble on fresh vegetables and drink lots of tea and coffee and chicken broth and diet soda-pops.

Q. When I lose weight, all sorts of wrinkles appear and my whole face seems to sag, and although I'm thinner, I look older. What can I do?

A. These signs of aging usually come from dropping the weight too fast; the body doesn't have time to reapportion itself. If you have weight to lose, do it *slowly*, no more than two pounds per week. After all, you undoubtedly *gained* the weight over a period of time; give your body the same opportunity to adjust while losing it.

Q. What do you think of diet pills and diuretics as diet helpers to lose weight?

A. I do not think it is ever a good idea to interfere with the chemistry of the body via pills or injections or whatever unnatural method is used unless absolutely necessary. Never, of course, without a doctor's supervision, but even then, only if all else has failed. Remember that with any drastic diet technique, you will face "normal" living when the treatment is over, and unless you change the way of life that brought you to such a state, you will go right back to where you started and will have traumatized your body for nothing.

Q. What can I do about backaches that come from a job where I must sit at a computer or typewriter all day?

A. As a writer, do I know *that* feeling! The answer is that you simply *must* get up from time to time and walk around for a few minutes—to the water fountain or bathroom, for example. One technique I have found helpful is to put my hands over the top of a door, feet barely touching the ground, and just "hang" there for a minute or so; you can feel the muscles in your back stretching. Another good exercise—if you are alone—is to lie on the floor on your back and alternately bend each knee (pulling it up with both hands cupped over it) up to your chest and bending your head down to meet it; this rounds the back and stretches it in the opposite direction of the sitting position. If getting up is impossible, take just a moment in your chair and round your back as much as possible, pulling in the stomach and hunching the shoulders forward, dropping your head. You will feel the relief immediately. You also have my sympathy—I go through this all the time.

On Makeup

Q. Is it true that women with puffy eyelids should not use dark eyeshadow?

A. Quite the reverse. Remember that dark recedes and light brings forward. Dark eyeshadow diminishes the appearance of puffiness, but if your eyelids are also wrinkled, I would recommend cream shadow. Also be sure to apply the dark color only on the puffy area (which is usually just above the crease line), and color the lid a medium shade to provide some contrast, so that the deep shade can be even more effective.

Q. I hate to use foundation. Is there anything else I can do?

A. You can get a natural color pigment called *Neutracolor* in a dark brown shade (at the drugstore) and mix it with your moisturizer or protection cream. This will give you some color with no more coating than your cream. You can also mix "bronzers" with your cream for the same effect.

Q. My skin seems to soak up makeup; an hour after I apply it, it seems to vanish. What to do?

A. This can be a difficult problem. Aside from the obvious answer of touching up your makeup more often, you might try using *dry* makeup rather than cream and using a water-based foundation, which is not as soluble.

Q. My husband insists upon the natural look, but my *natural* skin needs some help these days; how can I add color without his knowing?

A. First, be sure you know how to apply a complete makeup with ease, following the instructions in chapter 5. Next, read how to apply the "No-Makeup" look in that same chapter. In order to please both you and your husband, you must be more clever than ever. No *color* colors, only touches of pink at the end of your makeup in the places mentioned in chapter 5, blended well. *Blending* is the real key here. If all makeup is blended well both into the skin and into each other, there will be no makeup apparent on the face at all, and yet, you will *somehow* (!) look younger and more rested than you did the day before.

On General Beauty

Q. I love to wear pants, but I have large hips. What do you suggest?

A. I really suggest skirts that can much more easily camouflage large hips and stomachs. But if you must wear pants, make sure they are not too tight, not made of polyester, and it will help a lot if you wear an overblouse that softly covers the area in question, ending at or just below the crotch line. A self-tie on the blouse can also help to define the waist area (don't tie it tight) without calling attention to the wide hips.

Q. When my mother died, I was left a beautiful ring studded with twelve diamonds, but it looks very fussy and old-fashioned to me. When should I wear it?

A. Don't. Gem-piled jewelry used to be a status symbol and was always as tasteless as designer initials are today. Take the ring to a jeweler you are *sure* of—this is important, or you may not get back the diamonds you brought in—and have him dismantle the ring and make you something new . . . another ring with some of the stones and perhaps a necklace or earrings with the rest.

Q. Is there any product on the market that will make my nails grow?

A. Gelatin capsules or powder mixed into juice can be very helpful, as can protein supplements from the health food store. One very effective method for promoting growth is to massage your nails from base to tip (in a stroking motion) or even just press them—anything to bring blood to nourish the nail. Many nails do not grow simply from lack of good circulation.

Q. I love the braless look, but I am big-breasted. Is there anything I can do to look uplifted without a bra?

A. At the end of some fashion magazines, in the mail order section, you can find little half-cups that can be glued into place just under each breast for invisible uplift. Or you can make your own by cutting small half-circles out of a relatively stiff fabric and either gluing them on with surgical glue or taping them on with masking or adhesive tape. When removing tape, apply warm, wet washcloth to dissolve the glue; otherwise you could pull some skin off with your "no-bra."

Q. I hate the look of pajamas, but when I wear a nightgown to bed, it always ends up around my neck. Any ideas?

A. My first reaction is to say, "Don't wear either." But if you like something pretty to sleep in without the fuss, why not try wearing just the lovely top of shorty pajamas—the kind that look like a nightgown on top with little panties as bottoms and used to be called "baby dolls."

Q. What can I do for wrinkled hands?

A. Wash them well, but not too often, using a good hand cream each time and give them a defoliating beauty mask once every couple of weeks. Very often, "old-looking" hands can gain a youthful appearance immediately by simply ridding them of dead skin cells that have built up on the surface.

Q. I am quite heavy and can find no really stylish clothes in my size. What can I do to look younger and still fit my size?

A. Go to the maternity section of your department store or a specialty shop for maternity clothes. I'm not kidding. These fashions are designed for young (at least of child-bearing age) women with extra weight. You will be pleasantly shocked at how wonderful they can look on you—they have both style and room.

Q. I need to wear a girdle for my hips and stomach, but I end up with bulging thighs where the girdle stops. Are there any alternatives?

A. First, select a girdle of the lightest weight possible; the light Spandex materials are both effective and almost invisible under clothing. If this doesn't help, try an undergarment with legs that come down nearly to the knees; this will smooth out the thigh area. If you are not *too* heavy, my best suggestion is to wear a body stocking with hose attached, which will keep the entire line fluid without any stopping points.

13

WORK SHEETS

INDEX